ROBERT MANN

# MINDFUL BODY

# CALISTHENICS

*Achieving Physical and Mental Harmony through Mindful Movement (2024 Guide)*

Copyright © 2023 by ROBERT MANN

All rights reserved. No part of this publication may be reproduced, stored or transmitted in any form or by any means, electronic, mechanical, photocopying, recording, scanning, or otherwise without written permission from the publisher. It is illegal to copy this book, post it to a website, or distribute it by any other means without permission.

First edition

This book was professionally typeset on Reedsy.
Find out more at reedsy.com

# Contents

| | | |
|---|---|---|
| 1 | BOOK NAME | 1 |
| 2 | Chapter 2 | 2 |
| 3 | Introduction | 3 |
| 4 | The Science of Muscle Building | 5 |
| 5 | Is the Gym Really Necessary? | 6 |
| 6 | The Natural Calisthenics Body | 7 |
| 7 | The Importance of Muscles | 8 |
| 8 | Hypertrophy: How Muscles Grow | 9 |
| 9 | The Role of Hormones in Muscle Growth | 11 |
| 10 | Nutrition | 12 |
| 11 | Carbohydrates, Protein, and Fats | 13 |
| 12 | Ideal Sources of Protein | 16 |
| 13 | Calories In, Calories Out, and Building Muscle | 17 |
| 14 | Your Basal Metabolic Rate | 18 |
| 15 | Diet | 19 |
| 16 | Risks of Bad Diets | 26 |
| 17 | Rest, Recovery, and Consistency | 27 |
| 18 | The Importance of Rest and Recovery | 28 |
| 19 | Maximize Muscle Growth With Rest Days | 30 |
| 20 | The Role of Protein in Recovery | 33 |
| 21 | The Underestimated Importance of Sleep | 35 |
| 22 | Proper Exercise Selection | 39 |
| 23 | Compound vs. Static Exercises | 40 |
| 24 | Compound Exercises | 41 |

| | | |
|---|---|---|
| 25 | Static Exercises | 43 |
| 26 | Whole Body Workout | 45 |
| 27 | Pull Exercises for Upper Body | 46 |
| 28 | Pull-Ups | 47 |
| 29 | Chin-Ups | 48 |
| 30 | Push Exercises for Upper Body and Core | 49 |
| 31 | Push-Ups | 50 |
| 32 | Dips | 51 |
| 33 | Exercises for the Core | 53 |
| 34 | Leg Raises | 54 |
| 35 | Side Planks | 56 |
| 36 | Superman | 58 |
| 37 | Squats | 60 |
| 38 | Calf Raises | 62 |
| 39 | Master | 64 |
| 40 | Pull-Ups | 65 |
| 41 | Chin-Ups | 67 |
| 42 | Push-Ups | 69 |
| 43 | Dips | 71 |
| 44 | Leg Raises | 73 |
| 45 | Side Planks | 75 |
| 46 | Superman | 77 |
| 47 | Squats | 80 |
| 48 | Calf Raises | 82 |
| 49 | Your 21-Day Workout Plans | 84 |
| 50 | The Importance of Planning | 85 |
| 51 | Cardio Exercise and Diet Plan | 87 |
| 52 | A Note of Caution | 89 |
| 53 | Shoulders | 91 |
| 54 | Lower Back | 93 |
| 55 | Knees | 94 |

| | | |
|---|---|---|
| 56 | Positivity and Motivation | 95 |
| 57 | Pre-Planning Principles | 98 |
| 58 | Beginning with the Basics | 101 |
| 59 | 21-Day Plan: Four or Five Exercises Per Session | 103 |
| 60 | 21-Day Plan: Nine Exercises Per Session | 104 |
| 61 | Your Initial Progress | 105 |
| 62 | Cardiovascular Conditioning | 109 |
| 63 | Progression | 113 |
| 64 | Basic Level 1 | 114 |
| 65 | Basic Level 2 | 115 |
| 66 | Basic Level 3 | 116 |
| 67 | Transitioning to Intermediate Level 1 | 117 |
| 68 | Intermediate Level 2 | 118 |
| 69 | Transitioning to Advanced Level 1 | 119 |
| 70 | Advanced Calisthenics | 120 |
| 71 | Pull-Ups and Chin-Ups with Leg Raises | 121 |
| 72 | Horizontal Rows | 123 |
| 73 | Reverse Grip Horizontal Row | 125 |
| 74 | Diamond Push Up | 127 |
| 75 | Handstand Push Up | 129 |
| 76 | One-Arm Push-Up/Archer Push | 131 |
| 77 | and Parallel Bars Dip | 134 |
| 78 | Myths and Misconceptions | 151 |
| 79 | Conclusion | 156 |

# 1

# BOOK NAME

### MINDFUL
### BODY CALISTHENICS

The Ultimate Body Weight Training Bundle Pack to Build Muscle, Lose Weight and Increases Flexibility.

# Chapter 2

**Beefy Calisthenics**
Step-by-Step Guide to Building Muscle with Bodyweight Training

# Introduction

How would you go about developing powerful, defined muscles? Do you picture pushing and pulling weights with cables in a busy, filthy, noisy gym? How about dumbbells, barbells, kettle weights? That need not be the case. Rather, take a look at the amazing bodies of male Olympic gymnasts: they have perfectly formed bodies from head to toe and well-defined muscles that aren't overly muscular like the builds of some muscle-bound weightlifters. There is a simpler, safer, and superior method without the need for devices, gimmicks, or risk of injury to achieve the ideal body than pumping iron. If you want to discover how to get the physique of your dreams, you're in the perfect place.

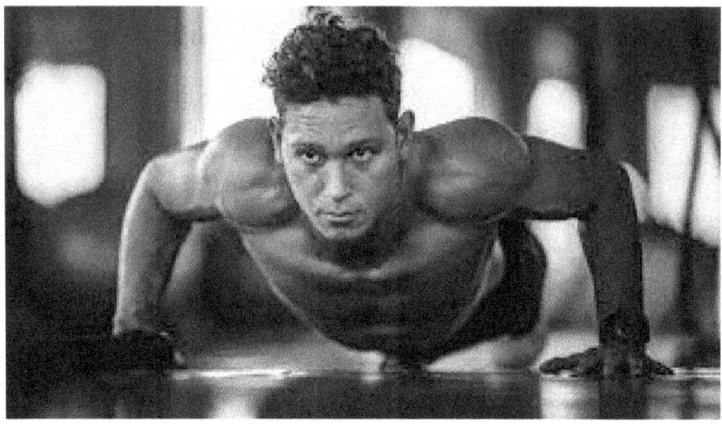

Men who desired to gain strength have long relied on a regimen of bodyweight exercises termed calisthenics, which predates the creation of fitness centers.

**Fig. 1**

# 4

# The Science of Muscle Building

Building larger, more impressive muscles is backed by research, and by adhering to a few fundamental guidelines, you may set yourself up for success in the form of observable, measurable outcomes. The secret to developing a fantastic body as you get noticeably stronger and start to feel and look better is knowledge. Knowing the definition of muscle, its composition, its growth, and its breakdown is the first step toward gaining knowledge.

As you will see in this chapter, exercise causes microscopic breaks in the muscle fibers that, when they mend, at the cellular level, produce new muscle. This is how our bodies are made to grow muscle. But in order to give the muscle fibers the right amount of stress, proper training is crucial.

## 5

## Is the Gym Really Necessary?

The quick answer is no, gyms aren't necessary, especially since calisthenic workouts allow you to tone your body and create muscle with just your body weight. You can get amazing shape without using machines, weights, or a gym membership. In addition, going to and from the gym requires time unless you live in an apartment complex or have access to a fitness center at home. Then there are too few weights and equipment, too many people, and the cramming.

Examine a few of the men who are lifting large weights in your gym. They frequently let go of the weights and can be heard groaning and sighing. You realize that's for your own advantage. These are conceited individuals who enjoy putting on a show. Is everything that

# 6

# The Natural Calisthenics Body

The question of what kind of muscles you want to create comes next after realizing that you don't actually need a gym membership. One option would be to get a home gym and start lifting weights there. However, since your bodyweight will provide you all the resistance you need for a naturally toned calisthenics physique, why spend money on weights?

# 7

# The Importance of Muscles

Whether it's when we see ourselves in the mirror after taking a shower or when we feel the warm glow from resistance training in our arms, shoulders, chest, abs, and legs, we can all feel our muscles. When we overdo an activity or any type of lifting, we are also conscious of our muscles since they are screaming in pain. But muscles are used for more than simply lifting, moving, sprinting, and jumping; they also have an impact on our general well-being, metabolic rates, and even lifespan. Beyond your objectives of gaining strength and muscle growth, having a healthy amount of lean muscle mass is essential to your overall wellbeing. Our bodies contain a variety of muscle types, such as the heart muscle (myocardium).

# 8

# Hypertrophy: How Muscles Grow

Each skeletal muscle is composed of thousands or even millions of minuscule muscle fibers, each of which is truly a muscle cell composed of connections called sarcomeres, the building blocks of muscle fibers that contract to genuinely cause movement. These sarcomeres, which house the thread-shaped contractile elements myofibrils, myosin, and actin, make up each muscle. Your brain stimulates the contractile fibers, particularly actin and myosin, inside the sarcomeres when it sends a signal to a muscle to contract.

Hypertrophy is the term for skeletal muscle growth. The process is intricate and starts with the myosin and actin fibers forming the sarcomeres, which then grow the muscle fibers and the muscle itself. Professor of physiology Len Kravitz, PhD, claims that:

Three components are involved in the development of muscle:

**1.Muscle Tension :** This is brought on by stress that is greater than what the muscles are used to.

2. **Muscle Damage:** This is brought on by extremely high

levels of muscle tension.

3. **Metabolic Stress:** It produces the "pumped-up" feeling by causing muscle cells to swell due to the influx of glycogen, an energy source. (To be clear, this pumping-up or swelling of the muscles is only transitory; the real muscle growth happens during the muscles' rest and recuperation phase following the exercise.)

# 9

# The Role of Hormones in Muscle Growth

Hormones are crucial for the growth and regeneration of muscle. It's likely that you are familiar with the important roles played by the male hormones testosterone and insulin growth factor. While the majority of the body's testosterone is used for different physiological processes, some testosterone is released during resistance training and can activate muscle cell receptors. In this case, testosterone's functions include promoting the synthesis of muscle proteins, decreasing the breakdown of proteins, and directing neurotransmitter chemicals to injured muscle cells to trigger the production of new muscle tissue. Insulin growth factor hormone transports amino acids, the building blocks of protein, to the skeletal muscles and promotes muscular growth and the release of glycogen for energy. Do these results imply that you.

# 10

# Nutrition

Eating is the process of nutrition, and the quality of nutrition depends on our diet, our ability to process and assimilate it, and the way it affects us.

The saying "You are what you eat" encapsulates the idea of nutrition really nicely. Naturally, things are not so easy. Our digestive tract breaks down food into its most basic components and digests it, allowing assimilation to occur at a deeper chemical level rather than at the level of cereal or Twinkies. Nevertheless, every meal we consume has unique nutritional benefits, calories, and other ingredients that our bodies must digest and respond to. Certain meals we eat might also have substances or chemicals that have the potential to be dangerous.

# 11

# Carbohydrates, Protein, and Fats

Calories are a unit of measurement used to indicate the energy content of food; one calorie is the amount of energy required to raise one gram of water by one degree Celsius. There are four calories in each gram of protein and four calories in each gram of carbs. Because lipids, especially oils, are made by nature to be stored, every gram of fat has nine calories. The main functions of lipids and carbohydrates are to supply energy, whereas protein helps to rebuild cells. Indeed, from muscles to red corpuscles in our blood, proteins rebuild every single one of the trillions of cells in our bodies.

Let's now examine the three basic dietary groups. Let's start with a standard, fundamental diet. Based on current bodyweight, the daily calorie need for weight gain, maintenance, or loss is determined. For example, an average adult male needs 2,000 calories per day to maintain a current, normal weight (i.e., not overweight or obese). The following diet plan comes from professional trainer and athlete Kathy Lee Wilson (2018), and she suggests that:

**Quality carbohydrates:**

Tought to make up 45–65% of the total calories consumed. You will be at the lower end of the scale in order to gain lean muscle mass and make more place for protein. The importance of carbs is often surprising to people, but we base this requirement on high-quality carbohydrates, which include the fruits, vegetables, whole grains, berries, and cereals found in the Mediterranean diet—more on which you'll read below.

**Lean proteins:** Can be as low as 10% or as high as 30% of the total calories consumed each day. You will be getting closer to the 30% protein amount if you are aiming for lean muscle mass. Just a portion of the problem needs to be solved by the protein that everyone requires to repair cells throughout the body, including blood cells, organs, skin, hair, and nails. When you perform bodyweight calisthenic workouts, your body breaks down skeletal muscle fibers and cells, which means it needs more protein to rebuild and repair them. Lean poultry, turkey, fish, low-fat milk, yogurt, and quality plant-based proteins including nuts, beans, seeds, grains, and cereals are good sources of protein.

**Healthy fats:** may make up 25% to 35% of your daily caloric intake. Since protein is essential for muscle growth, your fat intake may be lower, closer to 25%. The good news is that other foods in your diet, such as fish, olive oil, almonds and walnuts, avocados, and flax seeds, will provide you with the healthy fats you want for optimal health. It doesn't take much to attain the 25% target for healthy fats because fats provide more than double the calories per gram than proteins and carbs (nine against four).

In light of the aforementioned factors, your goal for the calorie ratio should be in the range of:

## CARBOHYDRATES, PROTEIN, AND FATS

- 45% of high-quality carbs,
- 30% of lean protein,
- 25% of healthy fats

What is the equivalent of these calories? Depending on how many calories you consume each day. An adult male requires 2,000 calories on average to maintain his weight, as we mentioned earlier. Recall that there are nine calories in every gram of fat and four calories in every gram of protein and carbs. Based on 2,000 calories a day, this translates to:

➢ **Quality carbohydrates :** represent 425 grams, or 900 calories, 45% of the daily amount.

➢ **Lean proteins:** represent 30% of daily consumption, or 600 calories (150 grams) per day.

➢ **Healthy fats:** represent 25% of daily consumption, or 500 calories (56 grams) each day.

(Search for the Fitness Calculator at the start of this book; you may download it and use it to calculate how many calories and grams of protein you need each day to gain muscular mass.)

# 12

# Ideal Sources of Protein

These foods provide adequate amounts of protein:

- Calories and Serving Size of Food Protein (grammes) percentage Every 150 grams
- Large eggs One (fifty grams) 70 6 %
- Rice, Barley, Peas, and Lentils
- Two ounces (dry) 180 7 5% Peas and Beans; 4 oz 120 7 5% Nuts (crunchy cashews, walnuts, and peanuts) 1 oz 170 8 %
- 8 oz of Skim Milk 80 10 8%
- Yogurt Greek (0% fat)
- 6 oz 100 19 14% Sardines 3 oz 200 22 15% Turkey, Lean Beef, and Chicken
- 4 oz 106 24 16%
- One can of tuna, 4 ounces, 260 26

# 13

# Calories In, Calories Out, and Building Muscle

As previously stated, one gram of water may be heated by one degree Celsius using one calorie of energy. Science has conclusively shown that calories in (ingested) and calories out (burned) determine how much weight is gained, reduced, or maintained. Although no two people metabolize, digest, and assimilate food at the same rate, physics dictates that if your caloric intake exceeds your caloric output, the excess will be retained as either fat or, more commonly, muscle, depending on how hard you work to build muscle.

You won't gain weight or fat when you up your protein or even calorie intake if you follow this book's instructions and complete the bodyweight calisthenic exercises.

# 14

# Your Basal Metabolic Rate

Your metabolism is at its lowest point when you are at rest, not moving or under stress; this is known as your basal metabolic rate (BMR). It speaks of the very minimum of calories your body requires to endure and maintain itself in the most undemanding circumstances. Consider your metabolic rate after spending hours in bed and doing nothing. You are aware that even while you are at rest, your body continues to need calories for involuntary processes such as breathing, heart rate, digestion, brain activity, central nervous system function, and, of course, muscle fiber repair.

While increasing lean muscle mass can enhance your BMR, it cannot be increased or influenced by exercise alone. Because of this, you may potentially burn.

# 15

# Diet

Though they may have various food preferences, nutritionists generally concur on the following fundamental idea: The healthiest and most optimal diet consists of actual food categories. Real foods: what are they? They're unrefined, nearly unaltered, nutrient-dense, and devoid of added sugar, refined carbs, and preservatives. There is also broad consensus that foods high in trans and saturated fats should be limited in diets.

The **Mediterranean diet** has been popular as the best diet in recent years for maintaining weight, staying healthy, and feeling better overall. There are many more methods to eat organically. Even if the Mediterranean diet does not particularly focus on gaining lean muscle mass, you are welcome to change the focus to protein that does so as long as you adhere to its rules.

The foundation of this diet is;

➢ **Plant-based foods :** give reasonable levels of wholesome, unprocessed carbs, healthy fats, some protein, and necessary vitamins and minerals. Vegetables, fruits, nuts, seeds, beans, whole grains, cereals, and vegetable oils are all examples of plant-based diets.

➢ **Animal-based foods:** are vital protein sources that include more of the necessary proteins for muscular growth than veggies. However, they ought to be eaten sparingly and only when the body is thin.

Foods derived from animals can include fish, eggs, and low-fat dairy products. All of these foods are excellent sources of protein and minerals.

Let's examine the categories of foods derived from plants that make up the Mediterranean diet in more detail.

1. **Vegetables :** are rich in vitamins, minerals, nutrients, healthy fiber, and even a reasonable amount of protein, despite having little calories and carbs.

Broccoli, bell peppers, and asparagus are among the vegetables that the Mediterranean diet promotes you to eat. They are low in calories and carbs and high in fiber, antioxidants, and vitamins K and C. Beets, carrots, Brussels sprouts, cucumbers, and kale all have these same nutrients. Though they are considered a fruit, tomatoes are rich in minerals including vitamin C.

In actuality, practically every vegetable you buy at the grocery store is a low-carbohydrate source of antioxidants, vitamins, and minerals. Aside from those, keep an eye out for Swiss chard, yellow squash, green zucchini, celery, cabbage, leeks, and onions. According to experts, a combination of colors is best for.

1. **Fruits and berries:**

S are sweet and tasty by nature, yet they are also nutrient-dense.

Apples are a good source of fiber, vitamin C, and antioxidants and very satisfying. They make a filling and healthful after-meal snack or the perfect healthy dessert. Vitamin B6, fiber, and potassium, an electrolyte, are all abundant in bananas. These same elements can be found in blueberries, which are also a good source of antioxidants.

Although they belong to the fruit family as well, avocados are rich in potassium, vitamin C, and polyunsaturated avocado oil, and low in carbs. Oranges, strawberries, grapes, and the majority of other fruits, melons, and berries are also excellent providers of fiber and vitamin C.

1. **Grains and cereals:**

have been a part of our history since the earliest hunter-gatherers picked wild wheat and, subsequently, when the first farmers started growing rice, rye, wheat, and other grains. Whole grains, which keep their bran, fiber, minerals, and vitamins, are preferred over refined grains in a diet rich in nutrients.

The most well-liked whole grains include brown rice, quinoa, and unsweetened whole-grain breads and cereals. These grains are high in fiber, magnesium, and vitamin B. Remember that "multi-grain" does not equate to whole grain; check the labels and limit your intake to whole-grain breads and unprocessed, unrefined grains and cereals. Oatmeal's soluble fiber and beta-glucan concentration are responsible for reducing LDL (bad) cholesterol. Regular oatmeal is higher in nutrients and only takes three minutes to cook, so choose that over precooked oatmeal Grains.

1. **Beans and legumes :** belong to the group of plant foods known as pulses.

Although we are most familiar with the dried kind, other types of pulses include peas and string beans. Beans are incredibly high in protein and other essential elements considering their small size. Pinto beans, kidney beans, chickpeas, black beans, navy beans, cannellini beans, and soybeans are examples of beans. Lentils and split peas are also included. Each serving of ¼ cup contains around 7 to 8 grams of protein (measured dry). You can start with dry or utilize the pre-cooked canned variations. (If utilizing dried beans, make sure to soak them beforehand.)

Beans offer complex carbohydrates, iron, phosphorus, fiber, folate, linoleic and oleic unsaturated acids, and protein. T.H. Chan School of Medicine at Harvard cites clinical studies.

1. **Nuts and seeds :** are a surprisingly good source of nutrients and are primarily utilized in snacks, cereal additives, and bread making.

Nuts are rich in fiber and healthy antioxidant oils. Examples of nuts include cashews, walnuts, peanuts (which are actually legumes), pecans, and almonds.

Protein, copper, magnesium, folate, potassium, vitamins B6 and E, and niacin are all found in above-average amounts in nuts. Research has demonstrated that nuts can help prevent cancer, diabetes, and heart disease. The well-known pumpkin, sunflower, chia, and flax seeds are among the seeds. Flax seeds, which have gained popularity recently, can be added to cereals and fruits to boost antioxidants, fiber content, and magnesium and calcium levels.

1. **Olive oil:** and the majority of other oils originating from plants are a perfect, advantageous source of essential fats.

Monounsaturated oleic acid, which makes up the majority of the molecular structure of olive oil, is an unsaturated lipid that has been shown in studies to be beneficial to heart health, particularly in avoiding the accumulation of LDL (bad) cholesterol, which can clog arteries (Joe Leech, 2018). Results also attribute olive oil's high antioxidant and anti-inflammatory content. It can lower your chance of getting diabetes, strokes, and Alzheimer's.

Use extra virgin olive oil, which is the healthiest and least processed type. Numerous other useful plant-based oils are polyunsaturated, such as soybean, sunflower, corn, and safflower. A few plant-based oils that are high in saturated fats should be avoided, including.

Let's now examine foods that come from **animals** and are a part of the **Mediterranean diet.**

1. **Meats ,** when consumed in moderation, are a great source of protein that builds muscle.

You should select lean meats, such as lean beef, which is an excellent provider of iron, lean pork, white flesh chicken, and white meat turkey. Take care to steer clear of meats that are loaded with saturated fats, as these should be avoided for both calorie management and cardiovascular health.

Meat portions ought to be smaller than you might imagine. The American Heart Association (2020) and nutritionists recoommend that a serving of lean meat should be three to four ounces, or around the size of a deck of cards. However, you might need to increase the portion size of lean meat if your objective is to gain larger, stronger, and leaner muscle mass.

1. **Fish ,** is a highly suggested source of important nutrients and high-quality protein. You should ideally have at least two servings of fish every week in your diet. Seabass, tuna, sardines, swordfish, mackerel, cod, and salmon are all great sources of protein. These cold-water fish have unsaturated fats and oils. Iodine and beneficial omega-3 fatty acids are also found in fish.

Studies have shown a correlation between diets high in seafood and longer, healthier lives with lower rates of heart disease, depression, and anxiety.

1. **Dairy,** goods, such as cheese, yogurt, and milk, provide sufficient amounts of vitamins and protein. You should restrict your intake of cheese overall and stick to choosing fat-free or low-fat milk and yogurt. As full-fat cheeses and cream contain a lot of saturated fat, try to avoid or use them sparingly.

Because the straining procedure eliminates extra water, Greek and Icelandic yogurts have higher protein levels than ordinary yogurts, which is why they are becoming more and more popular.

1. **Red wine,** is typically a part of the Mediterranean diet, and research suggests that moderate consumption is associated with healthier hearts and overall health.

According to certain research, those who consume red wine and other alcoholic beverages in moderation are healthier than those who don't drink at all or who drink heavily. However, prudence is suggested. For adult men, moderate consumption is defined as consuming no more than two 5-ounce glasses of wine, two 1.5-ounce portions of alcohol, or two 12-ounce servings of beer daily. Physicians recommend against starting to drink alcohol if you don't already.

You might be curious about eggs. Nutritionists currently rank eggs highly on the nutritional chart and suggest eating up to two eggs per day as a healthy food, despite concerns about the cholesterol content of eggs being voiced decades ago.

# 16

# Risks of Bad Diets

Over the course of millennia, humans developed to consume a wide range of natural, unprocessed, or barely processed foods that are rich in proteins, full of nutritious carbs and oils, and that provide the whole range of essential amino acids. These foods are known as the Mediterranean diet. They avoided eating items that were oily, fried, highly processed, contained artificial preservatives, had added sugar or other refined carbohydrates, or were high in trans, hydrogenated, and saturated fats. They didn't consume junk food, and we shouldn't either.

Consider the hamburger as an illustration of how food may have both positive and poor qualities based on their contents. Consider a hamburger made with only two basic ingredients: a whole-grain bun and 95% lean, unprocessed chopped meat. Lean meat is providing.

# 17

# Rest, Recovery, and Consistency

You can't achieve the desired slender body just by performing calisthenic workouts. Diet and rest and recuperation are equally crucial. Your ability to optimize muscle development and rebuilding within your daily, monthly, and long-term routines depends on your ability to practice consistency and discipline. The first step—possibly the greatest step—is mental as you get ready to start a serious bodyweight calisthenics program and are dedicated to reaching your bodybuilding goals: Your promise to follow the workout regimen precisely as directed and—perhaps more importantly—to adhere to the rest and recuperation schedule.

Would you think about getting back on the road tomorrow and completing another marathon if you had just finished one?

# 18

# The Importance of Rest and Recovery

You shouldn't undervalue, disregard, or treat recovery as an afterthought when it comes to your calisthenics routine. Therefore, before you even begin body weight calisthenics exercises, we want you to realize how important it is to rest and recuperate. It's normal to think that the calisthenics exercises you'll be doing are the only things that count. But in actuality, if you don't allow yourself enough time for rest and recuperation after your workouts, all of your hard work could be for nothing. Some athletes genuinely experience guilt on days when they exercise infrequently or not at all, but this is untrue because sufficient recovery time is required for your muscles, fibers, and damaged cells to heal.

**Overtraining syndrome:** is a potentially dangerous side effect of not giving oneself enough time to heal. Exercise physiologist and sports medicine consultant Elizabeth Quinn (2020) states that overtraining syndrome is caused by training beyond the body's capacity to recuperate in the online fitness publication Very Well Fit. Rather of increase, the outcome is a decrease in fitness and strength. Compulsive activity, lowered immunity (making the individual more prone to infections, colds, and flu), persistently tight muscles, aching joints, and a decrease in exercise performance—such as performing fewer push-ups and pull-ups than usual—are all signs of overtraining syndrome. A decrease in energy, irritation, sleeplessness, and excitement for exercising are possible additional symptoms.

You can check your resting heart rate as soon as you wake up every morning to self-diagnose overtraining.

# 19

# Maximize Muscle Growth With Rest Days

There are phases to recovery, and each one has an impact on how your muscles repair and relax. Short-term or active recovery is the initial stage of the recovery process that occurs in the hours following an intense resistance training session. During this phase, you can engage in low-intensity walking or light lifting exercises (such as housework, gardening, or hiking at a comfortable pace). You should be able to stay active without overdoing it the following day by continuing with these light exercises. Additionally, you'll be replenishing your energy, hydration, and protein reserves. Numerous things are going on inside of you during this active time of recuperation.

The muscles, ligaments, and tendons are being restored as a result of the stretched and damaged muscle cells you challenged during your workout substance.

➢ **How fast and how fully:** Your individual recovery capacity is determined by your genetic makeup and general state of health. The amount of time you need to recover also depends on how hard and long you trained in calisthenics. You also need to take into account how much downtime you get in between each session.

➤ **How often you exercise:** Every week is crucial. More rest intervals combined with fewer resistance training sessions can result in longer recovery times.

➤ **Your diet :** has a significant impact on consumption of protein in general. To maximize the repairs of muscle fibers and cells, a well-balanced, healthful diet rich in a variety of natural, minimally processed foods (the Mediterranean diet, for example) will provide the vitamins, minerals, antioxidants, and anti-inflammatories required.

➤ **Stress:** may interfere with the sleep-wake cycle by triggering the fight-or-flight response of the sympathetic nervous system and increasing the synthesis of adrenaline and cortisol, which raises blood pressure, heart rate, and breathing rate. Stress should be avoided at all times, but particularly while you're healing.

➤ **Rest days:** may refer to any day that you decide to relax and skip intense exercise. Instead of engaging in physically demanding activities, spend time with your family or engage in other interests.

Three days a week should be your goal for working exercise. Physical trainer Randy Herring (2019), who has over 40 years of conditioning, solid muscle growth, and training experience, suggests three excellent resistance workouts per week on the well-known bodybuilding website Barbell.com. Less than three could not be sufficient to give you the muscular body you want, and more than three could lead to insufficient time for rest and recuperation.

Three parts can be distinguished in recovery time:

1. Take a 30- to 90-second break during the workout in

between sets (a set is a continuous set of repetitions, or reps, such as 15 pushups without a break). The 30-90 second break should be kept in mind when switching between exercises, particularly if you are performing sets of the same exercise again.

**2.** Take a two to four hour break from any additional strenuous exercise, lifting, climbing stairs, or carrying heavy objects as soon as the workout is finished. Still, it's acceptable to stroll and engage in regular activity.

**3.** Avoid doing any weight training, heavy lifting, tugging, or pushing for two to three days after your workout. Now is the time for the major reconstruction and healing.

# 20

# The Role of Protein in Recovery

As we already know, eating plays a critical role in recuperation as well as in the development of a lean, strong body. A healthy diet can promote protein synthesis, which is the process by which amino acids combine to form chains of peptides, which in turn make complicated chains of proteins, as well as replenish energy stores and bodily fluids. Our DNA codes every protein molecule to repair muscles, ligaments, tendons, or any of the billions of other cells in our body. Proteins and amino acids are also needed for the synthesis of hormones and enzymes. Since protein is the building block of all of our tissues, organs, muscle cells, and fibers, getting enough protein in our diets on a regular basis is crucial to the healing process.

It really takes extra protein to make the repairs and contribute to the small overbuilding of the muscle fibers that results in bigger muscles because the damage to muscle cells is actually caused by a depletion of protein. And we need to get that protein, which is made up of amino acids, from our food. As you previously knew, you should strive to consume 30% of your calories from lean protein, which may be found in both plant and animal sources. Having enough protein on hand for recuperation also lessens the likelihood that the body would use healthy protein for repairs, which is a damaging process known as catabolism.

Athletes completing a hard training program can benefit from consuming twice the daily recommended amount of protein, or up to 2.0 grams per kg (2.2 lbs), according to research published by the International Society of Sports Nutrition (ISSN). For instance, a 165-pound person would need to take 150 grams of protein every day, either with a supplement or not (Kerksick et al., 2018).

It helps to eat a protein-rich supper shortly after your workout because you will be consuming more protein than you would normally get each day (30 grams, or around 150 grams) as a percentage of your total calories. For instance, if you work out before breakfast, have Greek yogurt, two eggs, wholegrain bread, and oatmeal with flax and nuts for breakfast after your workout.

Likewise, if you work out hard right before lunch or supper, eat a meal high in protein right after. Must you think about taking a protein supplement? Numerous powders and drinks made from plants and dairy can offer 15 to 20 grams of protein on average per serving. Athletes often depend on protein power to speed up their recovery from injured muscles, and Medical News Today reports that protein powder can aid in the regeneration of damaged muscles and tissues (Leonard, 2018). By promoting muscle protein synthesis, protein supplements used after strenuous exercise might expedite recovery and enhance performance (Leonard, 2018). If you're interested in protein and amino acid supplements, make sure to read the labels for ingredients and steer clear of companies that have a big list of names that sound chemical.

# 21

# The Underestimated Importance of Sleep

We may believe we are squandering time if we sleep in bed for eight hours every night. Many people are encouraged by this mentality to sleep less hours by rising early and staying up late. To extend their days a bit, some in today's digital age even carry their laptops, tablets, or cell phones into the bedroom. However, it turns out that scientific and medical evidence supports the age-old recommendation to "get a good night's sleep." We require about eight hours, and this is particularly important for people like you who exercise and are attempting to develop larger, more powerful muscles. Both your body and your brain require this entire night of sound sleep in order to repair and rejuvenate. Rest, it.

Additionally, your body metabolizes protein more efficiently and quickly when you sleep than it does when you are awake and engaged in physical activity. Getting a good night's sleep is crucial, especially after a strenuous workout when protein synthesis is most needed and cell damage is at its highest. The human growth hormones testosterone and melatonin, which are essential for cellular regeneration, are produced by your body when you sleep. Because your muscles are not working, the hormones force more protein to be produced than broken down, which results in a net increase in the size of your muscle fibers. However, protein is broken down more quickly than it can be rebuilt when you wake up and during the day and night. This is true even on days when you.

Stress reduction is one of sleep's additional advantages. In response to stress, our bodies increase the hormone cortisol, which in turn causes the muscles that oppose the growth hormone testosterone to receive bursts of energy-producing glycogen. It's the well-known fight-or-flight response. Stress has the potential to degrade muscle tissue and inhibit its regeneration. Getting a full night's sleep lowers stress and maintains high testosterone and low cortisol levels. Given that getting a full night's sleep is essential for maintaining both physical and mental well-being as well as muscular growth, how can we create and stick to healthy sleep habits?

Here's how to do it:

1. **Be Consistent** - Every day, go to bed and wake up at the same hour. Weekend exceptions should be avoided because the intention is to train your body to become accustomed to regular, sleep schedules.
2. **Don't Oversleep** - Your body clock can be reset by oversleeping, which makes it more difficult to wake up on time the following day. It will also be more difficult to fall asleep at the recommended hour if you oversleep.
3. **Don't Nap** - Although some experts recommend taking a short nap after lunch, even Winston Churchill rested, and naps help you feel less exhausted at nighttime. After lunch,

a cup of coffee is a better choice.
4. **No Caffeine in the Evening** -

Your body needs four to six hours for the caffeine to start to decline to the point where it doesn't keep you alert. That implies avoiding caffeine in the evening and right before bed.

1. **No Alcohol Before Bedtime** - If you do drink, get it out of your system before going to bed by drinking early enough. Just remember to drink in moderation. Alcohol reduces stage 2 REM sleep, or rapid eye movement sleep, during which the brain resets and dreams come true.
2. **Avoid Sleeping Pills** - You don't want to grow reliant on sleeping drugs because they can become a difficult habit to break. Certain sleeping medications, like alcohol, can obstruct dreams and the brain's natural reset process.
3. **No Digital Visitors** - Keep your laptop, tablet, and cell phones out of the bedroom. First of all, everything you read or see could be stressful for you, which would make it difficult for your nervous system to de-stress. Furthermore, the blue light emitted by these computer screens tends to interfere with our melatonin production, which is generally stimulated by darkness. Avoid watching television in bed for all the reasons listed above.
4. **Keep Your Evenings Calm and Relaxed** - The ideal time to avoid stress is right before bed. Steer clear of conflicts, confrontations, and tearful conversations with loved ones. Avoid watching violent TV or streaming movies in the evenings as these shows can increase your respiration and pulse rates, which can mimic the production of cortisol and adrenaline.

5. **Reduce Tension** - Take a warm bath or shower before bed if you are feeling stressed. Have something warm to drink; hot chocolate or warm milk work well in place of coffee or tea.
6. **Make Your Bedroom Conducive To Sleep** -

Your bedroom should have plenty of cool circulation, be quiet, and be dark. If there is poor airflow, think about adding a tiny fan, which will also produce a slight white noise effect. Make sure your bedroom is free of clutter to avoid falling in the dark.

Now that you are well-versed in the ideal methods for relaxation and recuperation, let's move on to the core of beefy calisthenics: bodyweight calisthenics exercises and routines. The first step in achieving your desired physical physique is choosing the right exercises.

# 22

## Proper Exercise Selection

Your calisthenics workout regimen will be based on the experiences of numerous athletes who have tried and tested every conceivable maneuver under a variety of circumstances. Think of the virtually limitless workouts at your disposal: pulling, pushing, lifting, bending, stretching, arching, extending, and compressing, to name a few. Think about using a lot, a little, or no resistance at all for each exercise. Think about the timing component, which includes the rate at which you execute each action, the quantity of repetitions, the number of sets, the interval between each set, and the exercise sequence. You will become proficient in all of these through the art of choosing the right exercises.

# 23

# Compound vs. Static Exercises

Exercises for calisthenics can either be compound exercises, which involve moving many muscle groups simultaneously, or static exercises, which only require moving one muscle group at a time. Compound exercises are often lot more effective than static ones at assisting you in reaching your fitness objectives.

# 24

# Compound Exercises

Multiple muscle groups are worked and challenged simultaneously during compound workouts. Exercises like the squat are examples of compound movements that target the quadriceps, calves, and glutes. A push-up is a compound exercise that works the glutes, quadriceps, shoulders, and abdominal muscles simultaneously. Combining two different or unrelated exercises at the same time, such a leg lift and lunges, is another kind of compound exercise. Leg raises alone would be classified as isolation exercises since they target only one muscle group—the abdominals. Compound exercises provide the benefit of exercising multiple muscles or muscle groups at once, although isolation exercises could be suitable when a particular muscle needs.

Compound workouts provide several advantages, including increased muscle work, increased caloric expenditure, improved intramuscular coordination, increased strength, increased muscle mass, and improved flexibility. They also help you accomplish more in less time. Additionally, as complex exercise increases heart rate and breathing rate, there are cardiovascular benefits. Experts advise making compound exercises the main focus of a workout since they view them as the pinnacle of strength training.

# 25

# Static Exercises

Isometric exercises, also referred to as static exercises, differ significantly from compound exercises in that they don't require movement—that is, there is no muscular contraction or extension. The muscles are neither squeezed or extended; rather, they are flexed and tightened. Because of this, only modest quantities of labor are being done, which results in a limited increase in muscle mass and strength. Although static exercises can simultaneously target many muscle groups, they do not fully test the range of motions in the muscles, hence complex exercises must be performed in addition.

Still, some static exercises can be incorporated into a bodyweight calisthenics routine. For example, the side plank is a bodyweight exercise that targets the anterior region of the deltoid, the quadriceps, and the abdomen all at once. Static exercises can also be utilized to work every muscle group in the body, including multiple muscle groups at once.

For people healing from illnesses or injuries that require low-impact exercise, static exercises are also beneficial. According to the Mayo Clinic, isometric or static exercises may be recommended to aid in the recovery of arthritis and rotator cuff problems (Salyer, 2016). Under some circumstances, such as while recovering from knee surgery, a shoulder injury, or a general surgical procedure, static (isometric) workouts may be a safer option than more demanding exercise, according to the online medical publication Healthline.com (Salyer, 2016).In summary, if your aim is to use bodyweight calisthenics to achieve outstanding shape and a physique you are happy of, then the majority, if not all, of your workouts should be composed of compound exercises rather than a single isolated or static exercise.

# 26

## Whole Body Workout

The greatest method for working out your entire body is to follow a set of prescribed compound exercises, often called circuit training, that focus on your lower body, core, and upper body. In this manner, it is possible to work different muscle groups in turn. For instance, it is preferable to work on your core, lower body, and then upper body again after performing workouts that target your upper body. One may ask themselves why a full body workout is required. Maybe all you want is a nice pair of shoulders and biceps. Of course, you want to look amazing from head to toe, but there are other benefits to a full body workout besides appearance. You'd want to.

# 27

## Pull Exercises for Upper Body

Pull-apart exercises strengthen and tone your forearms, biceps, back, upper body, and arms. To allow enough time for healing and rebuilding, it is recommended to execute these strenuous pull exercises twice a week.

# 28

# Pull-Ups

Yes, pull-ups—which you might remember from high school—are a great way to strengthen your upper body. Hanging from a bar with your arms shoulder-width apart and your hands facing forward while gripping the bar is how you accomplish a pull-up. After that, you pull up until your head clears the bar. You have a solid reason if you have ever found pull-ups difficult: they require you to lift your entire body weight without help. Think about how important proper form is when performing pull-ups. Focus more on your technique than on the number of reps you can do. It's possible that a coach or trainer told you to go "all the way up and all the way down,".

# 29

# Chin-Ups

These actions look just like pull-ups, with the exception that the hands are somewhat closer together and the palms are pointing backward. The additional work being done by the biceps in addition to the shoulders and forearms is one important variation in the effect of this activity. Just as in pull-ups, form matters in this exercise. You should be able to move your head over the bar, move all the way up, move all the way down, and not move too quickly. When you initially start out, pull-ups and chin-ups will be difficult for you unless you have been performing them frequently. The only way to become proficient at these two pull-up variations is to practice them regularly; there is no secret or short cut.

# 30

# Push Exercises for Upper Body and Core

Push-ups work and strengthen your shoulders, arms, chest, and triceps. They also enhance the strength and complexity of the central muscles that make up your core. Depending on intensity, push exercises should be done two or three times a week to allow enough time for healing and rebuilding.

# 31

# Push-Ups

Push-ups are a basic, dependable activity that most of us have performed at some point throughout our exercises, yet it is sometimes disregarded. It is worthy of our consideration and inclusion in a rigorous calisthenics program. Push-ups engage the arms, shoulders, upper body, core, and even the quadriceps slightly while using your bodyweight as resistance. They are a great compound exercise as a result. Push-ups specifically target the muscles in the chest (pectoral), shoulders (deltoids), upper arms (triceps), the stomach (abdominals), and the so-called wing muscles located beneath the armpits (serratus anterior).

The fundamental pushup is a terrific place to start, though there are more variations you can try. The back should stay upright, with the hands shoulder-width apart (no sagging!).

# 32

# Dips

A basic exercise that works the triceps at the back of your upper arms, strengthens your shoulders, and tones your core is the dip. Avoid doing push-ups and dips right after because they target the same muscle regions. Give yourself some time to rest in between by working out your upper or lower body.

Dips should be easy if you have access to parallel bars or any other equipment that will let you bend forward and lower your upper body. However, you can also perform bench dips in the following two ways:

1. **Option 1**

Two benches or chairs should be positioned parallel to one another and slightly wider apart than your shoulder. Position yourself in the space between the benches, put your hands on them, and advance your feet until you are almost sitting. Make sure your arms are fully extended. Directly lower your body as though attempting to sit on the ground. Even if you can't touch the floor, try lowering yourself as far as you can before getting back up. Try to complete the prescribed amount of repetitions.

1. **Option 2**

Place your hands on the front edge of a hefty chair or bench that won't tip forward while you sit down, leaving space for your body to go between them. You are now hanging your upper body in front of the bench by sliding your bottom forward. As much as you are able, lower your body straight down, and then raise it back up. Complete the prescribed amount of repetitions or as many as you are able to. You'll be amazed at how well dips work the triceps behind your upper arms, no matter how you perform them. For your next set of dips, reduce the depth of descent if you notice that your elbows are starting to hurt.

# 33

## Exercises for the Core

The network of interconnected muscles that stabilizes and governs the central torso of the body is known as the core. It consists of the muscles of the abdomen, the transverse abdominis (which are the broad, paired muscles on the lateral sides of the abdominal wall), the erector spinae (a collection of ligaments and muscles that rotate and straighten the back), and the lower lats on the left and right sides. An imbalance, strained muscles, and lower back pain can result from weakening or injury to the core muscles. Furthermore, the opposite of what you want with robust, rippling abs is a weak core, which will cause abdominal muscles to sag and result in a projecting waistline and stooped posture.

# 34

# Leg Raises

It is advised to perform this easy exercise to strengthen the lower back and abdominal muscles. Leg raises are said to be safer and more effective than sit-ups and crunches, which can put strain on the lower back muscles. Leg rises are a great way to build muscle in the abdomen, especially the lower abs. The secret is to do them slowly and thoughtfully, focusing more on technique than on how many you can do quickly.

Laying down on your back, you can execute leg lifts on a carpeted floor or a yoga-style foam mat. If neither of these are available, you can spread out a thick, cushioned blanket. Your legs ought to be fully extended forward. Put a folded cloth beneath your buttocks. Take a breath now and lift your legs to a height of approximately 30 degrees, or a foot and a half. After a brief period of holding that posture, release the air as you gradually lower your legs. Make sure, however, that they stay off the ground. Keep them slightly above the ground. For the required amount of reps, repeat this cycle. It's normal if you have to lower your legs all the way to the floor; with practice and patience, your strength will increase.

## LEG RAISES

Leg lifts combined with pullups or chin-ups might be a variant that results in a complex workout. In order to do this, you raise your legs to a horizontal position while pulling yourself up, then lower them as you.

# 35

## Side Planks

Crunches and even leg raises don't adequately engage the oblique abdominals, which are the focus of this exercise, which is helpful for strengthening the core. By strengthening the gluteus maximus and gluteus medius—the muscles we sit on—side planks also help to support your hips! Side planks spare your neck and lower back from strains and injuries, unlike certain other core exercises. Additionally, by improving balance, this exercise promotes ease of movement. Laying on your right side with your legs completely extended and your left leg directly on top of your right leg (or "stacked") from your thighs to your ankles is how you should start this exercise. It is proper to have your right elbow below your right shoulder. Release your left arm.

Try to hold the side plank for at least 30 seconds when you initially start out. Raise your left arm and point it toward the ceiling if you're feeling energetic. While maintaining the side plank position, try not to slump. Don't fall forward, roll, or keep the position for an extended period of time. Remain balanced and in the proper stance. Carefully release yourself from the

## SIDE PLANKS

posture when you feel too tired or incapable of maintaining it. While lying on your left side, repeat the exercise. This could be challenging when you initially start your bodyweight calisthenics routine, depending on your health. If raising yourself up on your right elbow proves to be too difficult, try pushing upward with your left hand as well. Do this two-handed again.

# 36

# Superman

Does "Up, up, and away" sound familiar to you? Imagine Superman, arms and legs spread wide, soaring through the air. You will use that Superman posture position to strengthen your core. This exercise strengthens the muscles in your back and legs, as well as the frontal and oblique abdominal groups and the shoulders. Although the Superman exercise appears simple, it may require some time and effort to become proficient in this crucial action. Because of its many advantages, yoga and Pilates practitioners frequently utilize it. This exercise works the entire core, shoulders, and legs while strengthening and increasing mobility to help prevent injuries to the upper and lower back. Sean Alexander, a.

  Stretch your arms fully forward along the sides of your head and your legs straight back as you begin by resting on your stomach on a mat or carpeted surface rather than a hard floor. Look down, not up or forward. Tuck your chin into your chest while imagining that you are Superman scouting the area below. By doing this, you will prevent straining your neck. Along with raising your arms a few inches higher, also lift your legs a few inches higher. Keep a steady pace and avoid moving too quickly. After a few seconds of holding the position at the peak of each rep, lower your limbs. Repeat after pausing.

The following ideas can improve performance and provide positive outcomes:

1. Raise only one arm and one opposing leg at a time (for example, the right arm and the left leg) if you initially find it too difficult to raise both arms and legs at the same time. Your ability to raise your limbs may be limited, but it will become better.
2. Make an effort to increase range of motion. Continue to breathe deeply and gently. Refrain from holding your breath.
3. As you raise your limbs, take a deep breath, and as you lower them, release it completely.
4. Refrain from overextending your arms and legs as this places excessive tension on them. Instead, when you complete the exercise, keep your limbs slightly bent. Exercises for the Lower Body It is impossible to exaggerate the value of powerful legs.

# 37

# Squats

This is the ultimate bodyweight exercise for the gluteus maximus, minimus, and medius, also referred to as the buttock muscles, and the quadriceps thigh muscles, which run down the front of our upper legs from hip to knee. In addition, squats strengthen the calves, adductor groin, hip flexors, and hamstrings (the muscles at the rear of the legs). It's also said that squats improve the range of motion in the core muscles. Since these are the biggest muscles in our bodies, working this set of muscles causes us to burn more calories than any other. Despite their importance, squats are a rather simple exercise to complete. With a little more effort required for the final few reps, you can easily do the majority of the required reps. However,

Start by assuming an erect stance and proper posture. To improve balance, place your hands on opposing shoulders and cross your arms in front of your chest. With your weight slightly on your heels, your feet should be shoulder-width apart. Now, approximately halfway down, steadily lower yourself into a squat position while maintaining a straight back. Although you have some leeway in this position, your thighs should be parallel to the floor. Lower yourself to the level necessary to use your muscles, but avoid going so low that your knees start to pain (little cracking in the knees is natural, especially as we age).

If your balance is poor and you have to walk forward or to the side, just lightly grasp a chair, table, or counter without letting go of any weight as you lower or raise it. You will find it easy to avoid falling over with some practice. To ensure that you retain your balance, avoid stooping forward and keep your posture straight during the exercise. Avoid attempting to go too quickly and instead keep a steady, gradual pace. When you get to the complete squat position, pause rather than immediately standing back up. Keep your breath moving. Take a deep breath and squat down. Every time you get yourself back up to standing, take a deep breath out.

# 38

# Calf Raises

It's likely that runners who press up against a wall or tree to warm up or cool down are extending their calves. Our calf muscles are vital to maintain strength since they exert a lot of effort into helping us stand and move forward. One of the simplest exercises to do, the calf raise works well to develop and shape the calf muscles while also reducing the risk of injury. Place your feet together or slightly apart, evenly distributing your weight. Elevate your heels to stand on the balls of your feet and toes. You should be able to complete calf raises without needing to hold on for balance if you are standing straight. However, if you require a little help, hold.

Place your front foot on a book, a step, or anything else that keeps your heels lower than your toes for greater calf muscle compression and extension. It takes more work to get the longer range of motion when you stand up. An additional way to do calf raises is to gently bend your knees while you rise and lower yourself. This causes the soleus muscle, which is smaller than the larger gastrocnemius muscle (the one that we recognize as the primary calf muscle) but equally important. Now that you have received this introduction to appropriate exercise selection, we can go on to the specifics, which will better acquaint you with these nine core exercises and allow you to.

# 39

# Master

You are prepared to master these nine exercises and create a strong foundation that will meet your goals of developing a muscular, strong body that you can be proud of now that you are familiar with compound exercises and the basic bodyweight calisthenic motions. Though every one of these nine calisthenics exercises was covered in length in the previous chapter, they are now offered here in a simplified style complete with videos and graphics so you can get started doing them right away.

➢ Use the links provided to get online demonstrations of the motions, stances, and exercises. To begin each quick YouTube.com video presentation, click the link found in the How section. (Most of the videos start with a quick commercial; to start the demo, find the little "Skip Ads" option on the lower right.)

# 40

## Pull-Ups

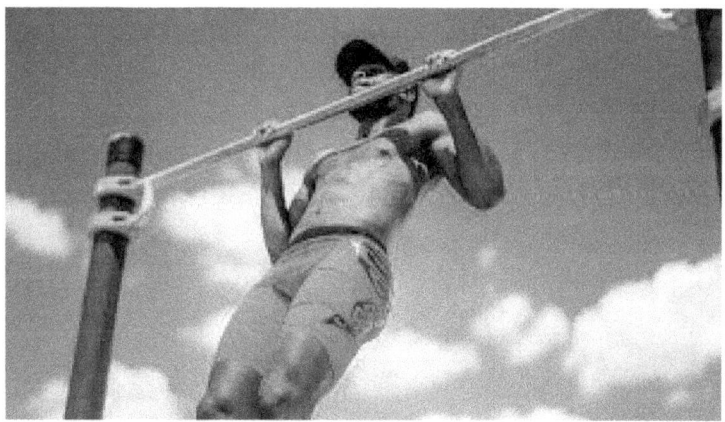

**Fig. 2**

**Where:** If there isn't a horizontal bar at your house, you can generally find one to use in a park or other outside space. The bar should be the same height as your outstretched arms. Pull-up/chin-up bars are also available for purchase; this is the only equipment you might need to acquire to complete this workout.

How Grasp the bar with both hands, palms facing forward, by reaching up. You should distance your arms shoulder-width apart. When your head is above the bar, slowly raise yourself. After a little moment of silence, descend once more. Stretch to the limit. Continue the pull-up cycle as many times as you can without jerking, kicking your legs, or failing to reach the plan maximum.

The video demo can be accessed at this link:
https://www.youtube.com/watch?v=eGo4IYlbE5g

**Result:**

This is mostly an exercise for the upper body. Your shoulders in particular, as well as your lower and upper arms, will be affected by the exertion. If the legs are worked by pulling or raising them throughout the pull-up cycle, then the core muscles, such the back and the abdominals, typically have to do some extra work.

# 41

## Chin-Ups

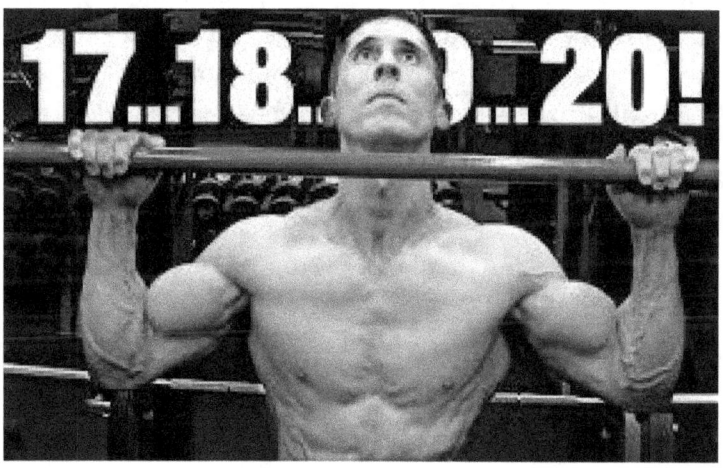

**Fig. 3**
**Where:**

The chin-up is the pull-up's fraternal twin and is executed using a horizontal bar that is at least arm's reach height under the identical "where/what" circumstances.

**How:**

With the exception of the grip, the motion is identical to pull-ups: the fingers and palms of the hands are pointed in your direction, and the backs of the hands are positioned face forward. It is possible to arrange the hands closer together than shoulder-width apart. The movements should be smooth, steady, and free of jerks, much like with pull-ups. Make an effort to reach the bar with your entire head—ideally your chin—and to stretch completely at the bottom.

The video demo can be accessed at this link:

https://www.youtube.com/watch?v=brhRXlOhsAM

**Result:**

With chin-ups, your biceps will work harder than they would on a pull-up, and as the bicep is worked up, you might feel a warm glow and heat (from blood and hormones building up). There will also be exercises on the lower arms, shoulders, and core muscles.

# 42

## Push-Ups

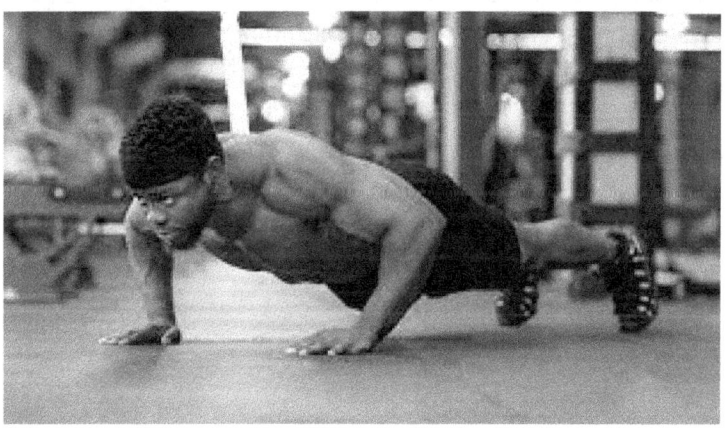

**Fig. 4**

**Where:** Push-ups can be done on any level surface.

**How:** Start with your body supported by your fully extended arms and your legs completely extended behind you.

To create a straight vertical line with your hands, elbows,

and shoulders, place your hands beneath your shoulders. Keep your back erect and slowly drop your chest to the floor without sagging. Reposition yourself to the starting position while maintaining a straight back. Continue for the intended amount of sets and repetitions. Once you've lowered all the way, don't immediately get back up, but don't stop either. Lower yourself to both knees if you're having trouble with push-ups at first and would like to make them easier. You can increase the difficulty of push-ups by decreasing the pace and taking longer to descend and elevate.

The video demo can be accessed at this link: **https://www.youtube.com/watch?v=IODxDxX7oi4& feature=youtu.be**

**Result:** This traditional compound exercise is excellent for strengthening your shoulders and straining your core.

# 43

# Dips

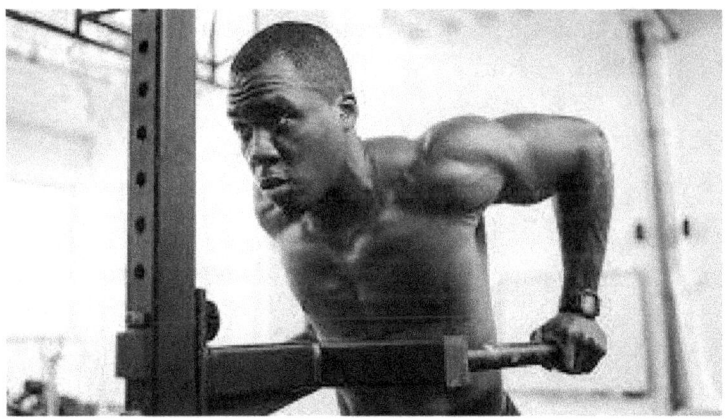

**Fig. 5**

**Where:** As demonstrated above, dips can be done at home utilizing chairs, boxes, benches, or counters. Just be sure that anything you plan to dip with remains stable and won't flip over as you go below.

**How:** To lower yourself between the two surfaces, place your hands on each of them. Raise your ankles and elevate your feet. To accomplish one rep, slowly descend as far as you can without straining, then raise yourself back up. One other way to dip is to sit down on a chair, bench, or countertop alone. Grab the edge of the surface and kick your legs forward to accomplish this. Slide your body forward till your bottom can pass in front of the surface while maintaining your weight with the palms of both hands. Bend your elbows to lower your body as far as possible without straining, then push yourself back up. As directed by the plan, repeat.

Here is the URL for the video demonstration:

**https://www.youtube.com/watch?v=isikOOF0W3k**

**Result:**

The workout will primarily target your shoulders and triceps, or the back of your arms.

# 44

## Leg Raises

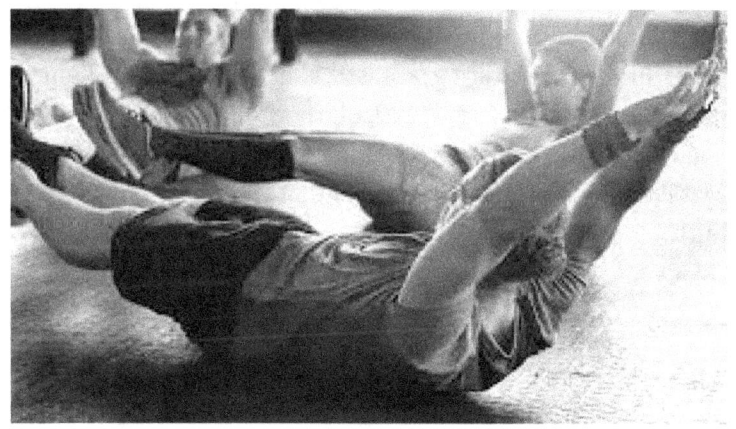

**Fig. 6**

**Where:** on the ground using a carpet or yoga mat (or any foam mat would do); a folded blanket can also work nicely.

**How:** With your legs completely stretched, lie on your back. Your hips should be slightly raised by placing a folded towel behind them (or, as demonstrated above, by sliding your hands beneath you). Lift your heels up to about 18 inches off the ground to start the action. The muscles in your abdomen should tense somewhat. At this moment, fully extend your legs so they point up toward the ceiling, then stop. Lower yourself slowly to the beginning position. Throughout each repetition of the set, keep your heels off the floor and lift your legs. While performing the exercise, try to keep your legs straight; if this is difficult for you, bend your knees. As previously indicated, you can.

**Result:** Leg raises are a fantastic exercise for strengthening the muscles of the core, particularly the lower back, frontal abdominal, and abs. Put a tiny folded towel beneath your head to relieve any strain if you discover that your neck is starting to hurt.

# 45

## Side Planks

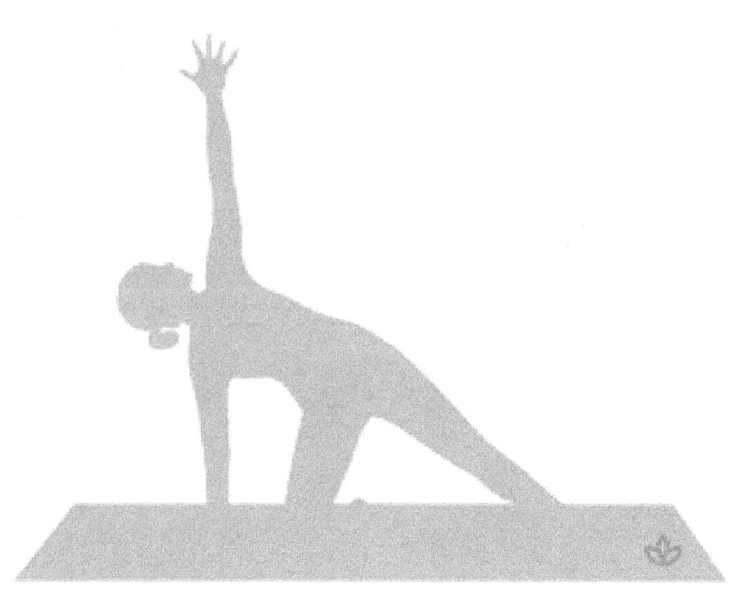

**Fig. 7**

**Where:** on the ground, supported by a folded blanket, carpet, or foam mat.

**How:** Place your left leg on top of your right leg after rolling onto your right side and completely extending your legs. Your right elbow and forearm should be squarely beneath your right shoulder as you support your upper body weight on them. Your left hand should be on your left hip. Now raise your hips while using your right forearm and elbow to support your body. Make sure your torso and legs are in a straight line. Raising your left arm and pointing it upward is one way to do this. When you initially start out, you might find this movement difficult. To help you lift your hips up in the air, you can use your left hand to press down on the floor. Additionally, you might discover.

The video demo can be accessed at this link:

**https://www.youtube.com/watch?v=NXr4Fw8q6oo**
**Results:**

Your glutes, which support the hips and enhance balance, your oblique abdominals, and your core will all improve once you can do this exercise, even just a little bit. You will also be working on your shoulders.

# 46

# Superman

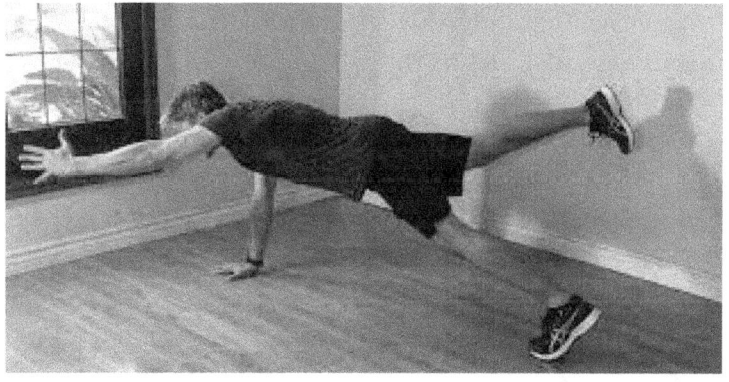

**Fig. 8**
**Where:** on the ground, helped along by a folded blanket,

carpet, or foam mat. Make sure you have adequate space for your arms and legs to fully extend.

**How:** Stretch your legs behind you with your toes pointed back, then reach as far forward as you can while keeping your arms against your head. Lift your arms and hands a couple inches higher. The same applies to your legs. The ideal position for your arms and legs would be with your arms lifted from your shoulders and your legs raised from your hips—this may take some getting used to. Raising one arm and the opposing leg, then switching the order (right arm and left leg, then left arm and right leg) is a temporary method for strengthening the muscles. Avoid arching the lower back by focusing on elevating the arms and legs.

The video demo can be accessed at this link: **https://www.youtube.com/watch?v=VUT1RHyMEuc**

**Results:**

This is one of the best exercises for strengthening the entire core, which includes the upper and lower back, front abdominals, and abs. It also helps with your shoulders, hamstrings, hip flexors, and glutes, as well as your upper arms and lower body. Just take care not to overextend or put undue tension on your lower back.

# SUPERMAN

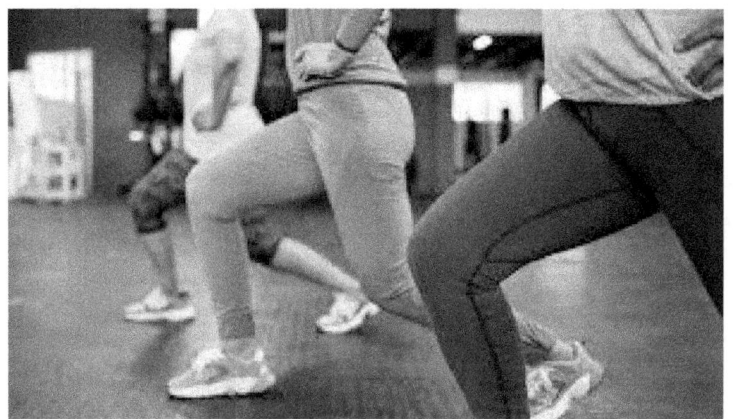

# 47

# Squats

**Fig. 9**

**Where** : Any hard, level surface. It's optional to use a table or chair to help with balance. You can also execute the move with a wall directly behind you to avoid inadvertently falling backward.

**How** : With your feet shoulder-width apart and your weight slightly turned back toward your heels, take an erect stance. Point your toes outside. Bend your knees and squat as if you were sitting in a chair while maintaining a straight back. Maintain a forward-pointing stance. When done properly, your knees should stay over your toes and not cross over. You can maintain your balance by extending your arms forward or, if it's still difficult, by resting one hand's fingers on a neighboring chair, table, or counter. It is only for stability; don't put any weight on it. Make an effort to bend till your thighs are in line with the floor. To keep your posture straight during the exercise, stay aware.

The video demo can be accessed at this link:
https://www.youtube.com/watch?v=aclHkVaku9U
**Result** :

## SQUATS

Warm quadriceps in the front of your thighs will be felt after a solid set of squats. Your hip flexors, calves, and hamstrings will all be toned by them.

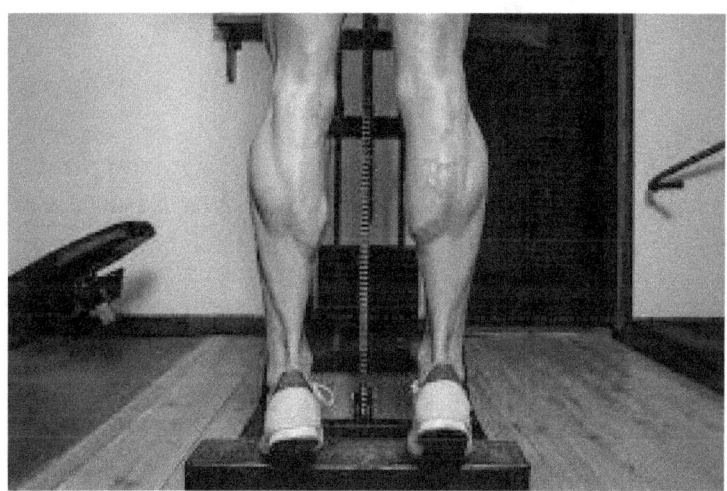

# 48

# Calf Raises

**Fig:10**

**Where** : Any level, firm surface or, if a longer movement is required, a step. It's optional to use a table or chair to help with balance. You can also do this exercise while standing one to two feet away from a wall, tree, or pole on a level area.

**How:** It just involves coming up on the balls of your feet and toes, stopping, then lowering yourself to the ground. You should feel the calf muscles contract at the top of the raise. Lower yourself all the way so that your heels are well below the level of the step and your toes if you are standing on a step with your heels extended. One way to make calf raises easier is to do them while seated in a chair.

The video demo can be accessed at this link: **https://www.youtube.com/watch?v=TZrBb5M1CdM**

**Result:**

Even though they are simple to perform, calf raises should leave your calves feeling warm and pain-free at the end of the set. It's time to create your customized training program, which is a timetable that determines your conditioning level and the course of the next three weeks. Every one of the nine bodyweight calisthenic exercises will have daily schedules that include repetitions, sets, and sequences. Because you will be switching up your muscle groups, you will work out most days of the week. Thus, one group works while the other rests. You will get the necessary downtime, but don't count on vacation time. Although calisthenics require daily dedication, as mentioned, intense sessions will be spaced out by two.

# 49

# Your 21-Day Workout Plans

Thus far, we have given you the fundamental knowledge of doing bodyweight calisthenics to gain strength, tone, and fitness. To ensure that you know exactly what to do and how to do it every day, the next step is to understand how to schedule your workouts. In this section, you will examine two 21-day regimens that will both jumpstart and sustain your progress over time. A nutritious, high-protein diet and cardiovascular activity are two more essential components of your conditioning that will be incorporated into your program.

## 50

## The Importance of Planning

Generations of trainers and physical therapists have been persuaded by extensive experience that an individual's ability to train and reach their fitness and strength objectives is largely dependent on their level of planning. If you've visited a gym or fitness facility, you've undoubtedly observed trainers guiding their clients through a set regimen of exercises on a daily, weekly, and monthly basis. Planning, when done correctly, guarantees continuous growth without placing undue effort on oneself or leading to injury. As a matter of fact, a lot of instructors think that pushing and pulling too hard and quickly during workouts might cause burnout, strains, or pulls, which can cause bodyweight training programs to be delayed by weeks or months.

Have faith in the programs that you will be following here to help you get the muscular body you seek while avoiding injury and overwork. Their creation has been centered around your prosperity and welfare. Don't undervalue the benefits of performing each exercise with just your bodyweight, even if you won't be utilizing weights or resistance devices. Yes, bodyweight exercises are safer than using machines, dumbbells, barbells, or cables. You can develop larger, more defined muscles with a recognizable "cut" musculature by following the recommended reps, sets, rotations, and rest intervals when performing the exercise correctly and with proper technique. You'll also gain strength and speed beyond your wildest expectations.

# 51

# Cardio Exercise and Diet Plan

Without the two extra components of cardiovascular conditioning and a sensible, nutrient-rich diet, your bodybuilding strategy would be incomplete. Cardiovascular activities that gradually increase respiration and pulse rates for an extended length of time have a solid medical foundation. These activities can be done in a variety of ways, including walking, jogging, running, swimming, biking, and using an elliptical machine. They should be done at least a few times a week. You will incorporate cardiovascular training into your plans because it is crucial for your general health and fitness.

If you did not spend too much time reading over the chapter 2 nutrition talk, you should definitely do so now. You should also go over chapter 3's explanation of the need of protein in your diet for maximum muscle growth. Maintaining a well-balanced diet will complement and improve the outcomes of your exercise regimen. Alternatively, you could disregard healthy eating habits, which could jeopardize your health and hinder your bodybuilding progress. You will not only be achieving your primary goals of looking good, feeling good, and getting much stronger by incorporating the life-enhancing benefits of body-weight calisthenics resistance exercises, regular cardiovascular conditioning, and a healthy diet; you will also be strengthening your resistance against obesity, diabetes, heart disease, and other diseases.

When considering things holistically, the most significant financial commitment you can make is adopting and adhering to a thorough exercise and food plan.

# 52

# A Note of Caution

The esteemed School of Calisthenics in the UK has based its training regimens on the theory of hypertrophy, which, as you may remember, is the process of building skeletal muscle fibers by subjecting them to extreme stress to the point where they are damaged and require repair by our bodies' protein ("Bodyweight training and workouts," 2020). The powerful tension that causes this healthy damage is, of course, provided by resistance training. The resistance must be just right—not too strong or persistent to seriously harm the mussels with rips, strains, and pulls—while still being enough to really work them hard. This brings us to some useful advice to assist avoid injuries that could keep you and your bodybuilding plan off the road.

It's critical to pay attention to your body, but not too much lest you overreact. Pain, however, is typically a warning sign that must be taken seriously. With practice, you'll be able to distinguish between the genuine pain that indicates significant injury being done and the typical burn that occurs when you're pushing through a few more reps toward the conclusion of a set. One major benefit of bodyweight calisthenics training is that you can only lift a certain amount of weight; you can't just add 20 lb weights to a barbell to increase the burden. Instead, you may increase reps and sets.

# 53

# Shoulders

Shoulders are one common location where resistance training (or any heavy lifting) can lead to injury. The rotator cuff is a collection of muscles that controls shoulder movements; if you inflict significant injury to it, recovery may take a while. Take extra care not to strain your shoulders beyond what they can handle. When it starts to ache a lot, reduce the tension and pay attention to any warning indications or severe discomfort. Exercises like pull-ups, chin-ups, and push-ups are fantastic for developing your shoulders, but be cautious of potential shoulder injuries. Additionally, your shoulder will be straining during side planks, particularly when you lift your hips off the ground to reach the holding position.

Excessive or repetitive use is another factor that can lead to rotator cuff injuries instead of harm from pushing or lifting too much weight. Baseball pitchers who require prolonged rehabilitation activities or, worse, rotator cuff surgery may be known to you. To put it into perspective, pitching seven innings can require seven sets of 24 repetitions, or more, of maximal effort (throwing the ball at 90 mph while also twisting your arms and shoulders to produce curveballs and screwballs). Your 21-day regimens will consider the need to refrain from overusing specific muscle groups.

# 54

# Lower Back

One such body part that is prone to strain and injury is the lower back, or lumbar portion of the spine. Do not arch your back when performing calisthenic exercises. For instance, when performing push-ups, maintain a straight back throughout the pushing motion and the stop at the peak of the exercise. The Superman exercise does require a small arching of the back, so proceed with caution. As you elevate your arms, shoulders, and legs, minimize the arching of your lower back. To relieve pressure on the lower back during leg raises, use your hands or a folded towel beneath your butt.

# 55

# Knees

The complex network of muscles, tendons, ligaments, and, of course, kneecaps makes up your knees. The muscle in your quadriceps aids in stabilizing the kneecap during motions such as walking and squatting. Ask a marathon runner about the symptoms of "runner's knee"—they include torn muscles, strained ligaments, and erosion of the lubricating cartilage under the kneecap—all of which can result from pattern and recurring injury to the knee. Squats are the one activity out of the nine you will be starting with that may cause discomfort or damage to your knees. Keep your knees from going beyond your toes and just squat as low as is comfortable.

However, in general, you should safely and progressively gain muscle size and strength if you adhere to the recommended increased repetitions and gradual resistance building that your 21-day programs call for. When resistance training is done properly, it can set up the body's machinery for muscle growth adaptations to occur when you push your muscles to withstand force, resistance, and newly imposed stress.

# 56

## Positivity and Motivation

Your mindset matters just as much as the workouts you will be doing. The first step is to set the objective of having a stronger, more muscular body and a healthier, more robust personality. The next stage, though, is to have the perseverance and self-control to reach and maintain your objectives. To put it simply, as legendary New York Mets player Tug McGraw memorably urged his teammates to believe in order to increase their confidence and advance to the World Series (indeed, they did). You have to have faith that your bodyweight calisthenics exercise regimen is effective in increasing your strength and bulking up your muscles on a molecular and muscular fiber level each day. Additionally, that it is occurring directly as a function of the time and

Experience has shown that most people find it difficult to begin a fitness regimen, be it a cardiovascular exercise, classic strength training with weights, or calisthenics. Experience also demonstrates that merely beginning a program does not guarantee sticking with it. We know of how many people who joined a fitness center, used it once or twice, and then stopped going? You're familiar with the justifications; "I don't have the time" is the most used one. Really? Does someone not have thirty to forty-five minutes to spare who wants to be in shape? It's difficult to think that the wonderful sensation after a workout and the advantages of gaining strength and muscle are not worth. the short amount of time. No, motivation is more important than time.

That all stems from "Ya gotta believe." You have to have a strong belief that this is effective and that you will reap the rewards of your efforts. Do you know about The Power of Positive Thoughts? When Dr. Norman Vincent Peale released it in the 1950s, it became a best-seller and continues to have a global impact on millions of people. The idea is straightforward and relevant to your fitness objectives.

You have to:

1. **Visualize yourself succeeding:**

Imagine yourself with the body you want and visualize it coming to pass. Envision doing every bodyweight calisthenics exercise and sense your muscles contracting and swelling.

1. **Think positively:**

About your capabilities and identity. Remind yourself again and time again that you are getting the muscle you have always desired. Don't let pessimism or failure-related anxiety control you.

3. **Minimize any obstacles:**

It could conflict with your training regimen. Consider the time you spend working out to be sacred, untouchable, and unaffected. Reject any potential setbacks during your workout by telling yourself, "I've got this."

# 57

## Pre-Planning Principles

While bodyweight calisthenics and weightlifting share many bodybuilding elements, there is a significant distinction in terms of creating tension to advance to more difficult muscle exercises. You just raise the weight being lifted while you do weightlifting. There's no need to adjust the rest and recovery periods, the number of repetitions or sets, or the timing of the motions. However, you maintain a same weight when performing calisthenics. You can only pull up your weight when performing a pull-up, for example—neither more nor less. This also applies to calf rises, dips, squats, push-ups, and chin-ups. You can only push or pull 165 pounds if you weigh 165 pounds. Consequently, several factors must come.

To start, let me clarify some terminology:

**1.** One whole exercise cycle is referred to as a **rep** (repetition). Consider the single push-up movement that goes up and down. Most of the exercises will likely require you to perform six to twelve repetitions at first.

**2.** A group of repetitions done in a single sequence is called a set. Thus, one set of push-ups is equal to your six repetitions, for example.

Initially, you should perform three to five sets.

**3.** The term **"rest"** describes the 30- to 90-second break that occurs between sets.

**4.** The amount of days that pass between a body group's workouts is called recovery. For instance, taking a two-day break between upper-body workouts and targeting different body parts during those two.

Now, here's how to increase the level of difficulty and muscle strain throughout the workouts without adjusting your own weight:

**1.** The quantity of sets and repetitions can be increased. For instance, going from six to ten to twelve reps. Alternatively, going from three to five to six sets.

**2.** The intervals of time between sets can be shortened. For instance, you might take a 60- or 30-second break rather than a 90-second one.

**3.** You can move more slowly, which makes the movements more tense. Take 10 seconds to lower and ten seconds to push back up when doing push-ups, for instance (try it; it's astonishing).

Some of the variations we covered earlier can also be included. As you progress, you can adjust the difficulty of a push-up, for instance, by adjusting the distance between your hands. Another option is to change your body angle and do a pike push-up, which puts more strain and pressure on your shoulders and upper chest. Alternatively, there are the more difficult pull-ups, such as the Korean dips, one-arm pull-ups, and one-arm push-ups. In the advanced plan, you can choose to try these or to continue with the simpler exercises, where you slow down and increase the repetitions and sets. You can choose to put on more weight to your body. Wearing a weighted vest, for instance, can add 20 pounds while you are.

The healing period is the one variable that you will not be altering. In most situations, a full two days are needed to allow for the necessary protein-based muscle repairs. This is especially important when the exercises get harder. Your goal is to increase the tension in every muscle in your body by combining various body parts while performing bodyweight difficult exercises. For this reason, calisthenics are more advantageous than machine training's pushing and pulling motions and the more solitary movements done with weights.

# 58

## Beginning with the Basics

The three primary muscle groups that each of the 21-day regimens targets are the lower body's quadriceps, hamstrings, calves, and hip flexors; the upper body's arms and shoulders; and the core's abdominals, back muscles, and side muscles. The nine exercises that you are now familiar with are included in the plans; as you advance, you can make changes to the form, technique, and timing of each exercise. Your plan's exercise sequence is designed to space out related muscle groups. You wouldn't want to do leg raises right after a set of squats or three sets of pull-ups followed right away by three sets of chin-ups. But you can change the sequence to fit your needs as long as you follow through.

You can work out with bodyweight calisthenics two or three days a week, or even more frequently, like five or six days. It matters how these two extremes differ from one another.

1. **Two or three** You will only do the nine exercises for the necessary reps, sets, cycle periods, and set intervals two or

three days a week if you undertake bodyweight calisthenics workouts. Put another way, you'll engage in longer, more intense exercises but with fewer training sessions overall. Over the course of the 21-day regimen, the two or three workouts per week add up to seven tough workout days.

2. **Four or five** Exercise days per week could be favored for people who enjoy doing calisthenics exercises nearly every day. The training regimen for that choice rotates between two groups: Group 1 performs five exercises, and Group 2 performs four exercises. With this choice, you will work out with calisthenics four or five times a week, or 14 times throughout the course of the 21-day regimen.

# 59

# 21-Day Plan: Four or Five Exercises Per Session

The nine exercises are split into two groups of four or five exercises per session for the duration of this 21-day regimen.

\* The number of seconds needed to finish a movement is called a cycle. For instance, a pull-up cycle consists of the movements of pulling up and lowering down, whereas a Superman cycle involves maintaining the position. The 21-day schedule for the two groups is depicted in the chart below. There are 14 training days and 7 rest/recovery days in this plan. Each group is separated by two days since the groups are done one after the other, with one day set aside for rest and recovery.

    The 21-day schedule for the two groups is depicted in the chart below. There are seven rest/recovery days and fourteen workout days in this schedule. Each group is separated by two days since the groups are conducted one day after the other, and then there is a day of rest or recovery in between.

# 60

## 21-Day Plan: Nine Exercises Per Session

Using a one-day-on, two-day-off schedule, all nine exercises are completed in a single session.

The nine exercises will be performed in the following chart in accordance with the 21-day timetable. As said, the 21-day program in this plan includes seven days for exercise and fourteen days for relaxation and recuperation.

# 61

## Your Initial Progress

You are now prepared to begin. The first thing you should do is decide if you would rather follow a schedule that calls for four to five workouts a week or one that allows you to exercise fewer days. You are more than welcome to test any timetable to determine if it suits your needs or not. Whichever schedule you go with, be sure you are having enough time to relax and recuperate in between workouts. The next thing you should do is try to stick to the suggested reps, sets, and timing. However, as we are all different, you may find that in the beginning of your training, fewer is better for you. Or you may discover that doing more comes naturally to you. More repetitions at a slower pace are possible.

About your early progress, you're hopeful that your ambitious bodyweight calisthenics routine would live up to your high standards. You won't be disappointed, so don't worry. That is, provided you keep in mind the value of dedication and give your all to your bodybuilding objectives. First and foremost, select some choices that will ease you into your workouts and keep them on schedule for the first 21-day plan in order to make sure you stick to it.

The following are some important things to think about when you start your selected 21-day plan:

1. **Where?**

The ideal space for your workout regimen is a room or area in your house with the necessary capacity as well as useful features or fittings. Think about: Does the room offer side planks, leg lifts, and flooring to cushion you when you're Superman? If not, do you have a blanket that can be folded into a cushion or a yoga mat? Regarding privacy, what say you? Distractions should be avoided if you want to be able to concentrate on your motions and feel your muscles contracting. It could be more comfortable for you if no one else watches you work out or says anything.

Even though your house could have enough room, you might need to go somewhere else to get a bar where you can perform pull-ups and chin-ups. It would be fantastic to have your own chin-bar, though. You can avoid conflict with roommates, friends, spouses, and partners by using one of these, which are safe to use and most of which can be swiftly put up and taken down. Online, there are a plethora of possibilities for chinning bars. To get started, simply type "chinning bar doorway" on Google. You're not just limited to your house; you might be able to utilize a bar or some equipment, like monkey bars, at a neighboring playground or park. This also holds true for the structures you can employ for dip workouts.

2. **When?**

Whether or not you continue with your bodybuilding calisthenics program can be greatly influenced by the time of day and days that you choose to train. Consider the timing carefully before making a decision. You must decide on one time of day and adhere to it. For instance, it's ideal to exercise first thing in the morning, preferably before breakfast or, if time permits, before lunch. Try exercising before supper if you are a slow starter and find that working out before breakfast or lunch doesn't work for you. However, avoid working out right before bed or right after eating.

Make a commitment to the time that suits you best. Telling yourself you'll work out early in the day and then deciding to "get to it later" is a mistake. Most likely, you won't. Commitment and consistency are crucial for reaching your fitness objectives. The days you choose to work out also apply to this. You don't have to wait until Monday to begin the 21-day program, but once you do, you must honor the "off" days for rest and recovery and the "on" days for exercise. Things do occasionally come up, of course, but if you miss a day, make up for it the next day. Rest is crucial, as we've stressed, so taking an extra day off is OK.

1. **Being Inclusive**

It's vital to complete all nine of these exercises, not just some, as they have been carefully chosen to ensure that your entire body will be pushed, developed, and built-up during your initial program. Refrain from focusing only on your upper body, such as your shoulders, triceps, and biceps, just because you have amazing muscles there. Give your entire core the same amount of focus as you do your lower body.

When you give each of the nine exercises equal attention, your muscles create an interactive network that works in concert, creating a synergistic impact. Every exercise works a variety of muscle groups and locations. Although the arms and shoulders may receive a lot of attention during pull-ups and chin-ups, your chest, abdomen, and upper back are also tense.

1. **Form and Intensity**

Make sure you adhere to the guidelines on how to complete the nine activities in chapters 4 and 5. Our goal in creating these instructions was to assist you in completing them accurately and completely. Don't forget to view the demo videos. Furthermore, even though the information supplied here is thorough and extensive, don't hesitate to conduct your own research as there are a ton of different demonstrations available online. You should complete every activity accurately and completely—no short cuts or cheating. When performing push-ups, you should go all the way down and back up while maintaining a straight back and pausing briefly at the top and bottom positions. Make sure you're doing it correctly. Likewise with pull-ups.

And don't rush through it. To ensure the right amount of tension is felt, watch your speed and perform the actions more slowly than quickly. One of the better methods to increase the difficulty of the workouts without adding more weight as you advance in the upcoming weeks and months is to slow down the movements. However, even in the early stages, go slowly.

As you descend into each squat, pull up and lower down, or drop and raise again, feel the tension in your body. You can be sure that your muscles are getting enough work to undergo hypertrophy by moving slowly.

# 62

## Cardiovascular Conditioning

The main goal of aerobics, or cardiovascular conditioning, is to increase your heart rate and maintain it there for an extended amount of time. You're definitely aware of it because you see runners everywhere, as well as folks using ellipticals, treadmills, pedaling and spinning bicycles, and swimming laps. When articles started to highlight the health advantages of exercise in the 1970s, there was a general interest in cardio. Millions of people of all ages were not running marathons prior to that time, nor had you ever seen anyone jogging on the streets. There were very few fitness centers, and the focus was nearly entirely on weightlifting in those that did exist.

To benefit from cardiovascular conditioning, do you need to train to run 26.2 miles and become a marathoner? No, there are plenty of less demanding and time-consuming alternatives to meet your weekly need for cardiovascular activity. You can utilize an elliptical machine or ski simulator, ride an indoor or outdoor bike, swim laps, or walk or jog at a moderate pace outside or on a treadmill. Make sure the activity is heart-pumping and rhythmic, and that you can maintain it for a minimum of 15 to 20 minutes (preferably, 30 minutes or longer).

We'll address your inquiries regarding the advantages of aerobic exercise below, and you can discover how to begin implementing an.

### 1. What are the health benefits of cardio exercise?

There is constant coverage in the media regarding the possibility of cardiovascular exercise to prevent disease. It's impossible to ignore the innumerable articles, health reports, and TV shows that stress how important it is to get up and move, boosting your heart rate and taking deep breaths for at least twenty minutes. Cardiovascular exercise has been linked to a reduction in the incidence of heart attacks and strokes by reducing the accumulation of arterial plaque and lowering high blood pressure, according to an ongoing stream of new research and clinical trials. Because cardio exercise improves insulin resistance and lowers blood sugar, it is also thought to prevent type 2 diabetes. Additionally, it might prevent digestive and respiratory issues and perhaps lower the chance of some types of cancer.

### 1. Does cardio help with weight control?

In America, one-third of people are considered overweight, while another one-third is obese. These divisions are predicated on body mass index levels, which account for gender, height, and weight. However, as cardio exercises burn a lot of calories, you can reduce your weight to a healthful level with cardio training. 400–500 calories can be burned during a vigorous 30- to 45-minute aerobic activity, which helps reduce excess weight and keep it off.

Your body uses carbohydrates (in the form of glycogen) for energy, so don't worry about burning off protein; if that energy runs low (like during a long run), your body will burn fat.

1. **Does cardio provide psychological benefits?**

The hormone that causes the well-known "runner's high," beta-endorphins, can be released during cardiovascular exercise. It has a medically proven impact that reduces anxiety and sadness as well as tension and stress. By this point, you probably want to know if performing intense calisthenics exercises can release beta-endorphins. Most likely, particularly if the exercise is done quickly. However, it appears that a cardio workout done at a consistent, high intensity is more successful at producing the runner's high. The physical and mental benefits build up when cardio and calisthenics are done at the same training session.

By growing the hippocampus, the area of the brain that controls emotion, aerobic exercise is also said to elevate mood. Additionally, it helps support restful sleep. Calisthenics and aerobics work together to increase brain plasticity, which enhances memory and learning capacity.

1. **Will cardiovascular conditioning help you to live longer?**

Cardiovascular fitness may extend your life, as it is associated with the prevention or delayed development of numerous life-threatening illnesses and ailments. To be objective, though, life is full with uncertainties, particularly in light of the significant influence that our genetic profiles have. Doing your best to increase the odds and give your body a fighting chance to survive and thrive for as long as possible is the responsible approach. Maintaining good cardiovascular health is believed by many marathoners to not only add years to your life but also increase the quality of those years.

**5. Do you need a doctor's approval?**

Medical and fitness experts advise you to speak with your doctor before starting any intense exercise, particularly if it has been a year since your last comprehensive physical check.

It's a good idea to get your heart and circulatory system examined, and chances are good that you'll be told to start slowly, ease into it, and gradually increase the intensity of your cardio and calisthenic training. During aerobic exercises, pay attention to your body's warning signals. Pain in your left arm, chest, or shoulder may indicate that your heart's blood flow is being restricted or obstructed, similar to the symptoms of angina. If that occurs, stop working out and give your.

**6. How much cardio exercise do you need?**

Most people agree that brisk walking or jogging, biking, using an elliptical, or swimming for at least three days a week is acceptable, but four or more days is preferred.

A total of 150 minutes each week is a reasonable baseline if the pace is moderate. A decent starting point is 75 to 100 minutes per week if the pace is brisk, using deeper breathing and increasing heart rate. However, some intense exercisers aim for 300 minutes a week. When you're in good shape, interval training—which consists of short bursts of speed and/or increasing incline—can improve the quality of your cardio workout. You should be exerting a lot of effort during the 20 to 40-second interval.

# 63

# Progression

Your calisthenics workout plan's main goal is to get you started quickly and simply so that you can progress to more intense levels later on. You will go through two intermediate levels after working through three basic levels, and then move on to the first advanced level. It is up to you to decide when to advance to a harder degree of intensity or a more intricate exercise movement. Your assessment of your level of expertise, your ability to execute each exercise correctly (with good form), your ability to finish the recommended number of repetitions and sets, and your willingness to adhere to the suggested timing for each movement cycle and rest period in between sets are all important factors to take into account.

# 64

# Basic Level 1

Here's where you're going to start: Day 1 of Week 1's Basic Level 1. This is the 21-day schedule from the previous chapter, when you complete all nine exercises in a single session, following a one-day-on/two-days-off cycle. For every 21-day cycle, this schedule offers seven days for exercise and fourteen days for relaxation and recuperation. Think of this as the base upon which you will build your progress over the next few weeks and months.

Begins Week 1
   Day 1

# 65

# Basic Level 2

You should be prepared to work a little harder and move on to Basic Level 2 after around two weeks of studying Basic Level 1. Depending on personal success, this level starts in either week three or week four and involves increasing the reps for most exercises. The cycle timing is prolonged, but the side plank stays the same at one rep each side. For every exercise, there are no modifications to the number of sets or length of rest interval between sets.

**Begins Week 3 or 4**
**Day 22 or 29**

# 66

## Basic Level 3

Depending on personal development, either week six or week seven can see the start of Basic Level 3. All of the exercises have the same amount of repetitions, but each exercise has a longer cycle time. Extending the duration of each up-and-down or down-and-up workout will undoubtedly make it feel harder. Sets and the interval in between them remain unchanged.

Begins Week 6 or 7
  Day 43 or 50

# 67

# Transitioning to Intermediate Level 1

You should have mastered Basic Level 3 by now, and week 10 will mark the start of the move to Intermediate Level 1. For the majority of the exercises here, the rep count goes up and the interval between sets gets shorter. The cycle timing is lengthened, but side planks stay at one rep each side. The number of sets and cycle time remain unchanged
  Begins Week 10
  Day 71

# 68

# Intermediate Level 2

Week 13 is when Intermediate Level 2 starts. For every exercise, there is no variation in the amount of repetitions; however, for certain exercises, the cycle time is prolonged. Sets and the interval in between them remain unchanged. The extended cycle times should definitely increase the difficulty of the exercises.

Begins Week 13

Day 92

# 69

# Transitioning to Advanced Level 1

You should be prepared to start Advanced Level 1 if you have been following the training routine and making progress through the Basic and Intermediate Levels. Remain calm and take your time repeating a cycle if you feel that you are not quite ready and need additional time at one of the Intermediate Levels. You should move at your own pace; there's no urgency. Recall that no two people will develop their muscles and strength at the same pace because we are all unique. Starting in week 16, Advanced Level 1. For every exercise, the number of sets increases from three to four, but the rep counts and cycle times remain the same.

Begins Week 16

Day 113

# 70

# Advanced Calisthenics

You could feel prepared to incorporate compound versions of the current nine exercises into your routine and/or take on more challenging versions of the exercises after finishing the 18-week Basic Level, Intermediate Level, and Advanced Level 2 plan. You start training for maximum results by pushing your body and mind at Advanced Level 2 and up.

# 71

# Pull-Ups and Chin-Ups with Leg Raises

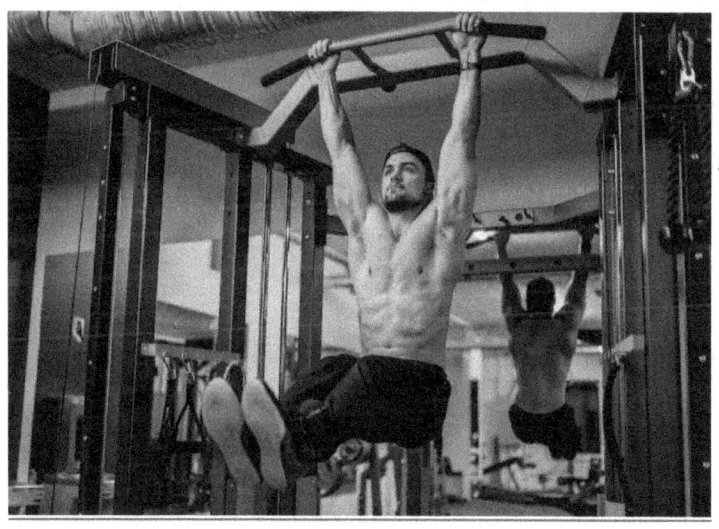

Fig. 11
**Where:**
For this exercise, just like a standard pull-up or chin-up,

you'll need a horizontal bar that's the same height as your outstretched arms.

**How:**

This is a compound exercise that works two different muscle groups at once to enhance the amount of work done in a given amount of time and to challenge and engage them. When performing pull-ups, place both hands on the bar, palms facing forward, and place your arms shoulder-width apart. In order to perform chin-ups, turn your palms facedown. Raise your legs and fully extend them till they are parallel to the ground, if at all feasible, as you steadily pull yourself upward (or lift as far as you can). As soon as your head touches the bar, stop and carefully lower yourself back down. At the same time, gradually lower your legs to the vertical (downward position). While performing the pull-up or chin and leg lift cycle, repeat it as many times as you can.

By bringing your knees up to your chest, like in the picture above, rather of fully extending your legs wide, you can make leg raises easier. To increase the difficulty, keep your legs completely extended and parallel to the floor while you raise and lower yourself for the necessary number of cycles.

The video demo can be accessed at this link:

**https://www.youtube.com/watch?v=QyVq50UBpss**

**Result:**

Even though this is mainly an upper-body workout, the leg lifts work the quadriceps, hip flexors, back, stomach, and core muscles.

# 72

# Horizontal Rows

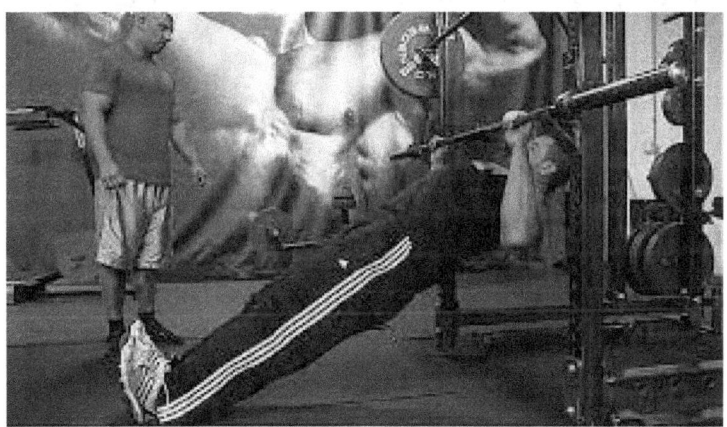

**Fig. 12**

**Where:**

At home, horizontal rows can be accomplished using common furniture, a lowered chinking bar, or even just a sheet in a doorway (as demonstrated above).

**How:**

One way is to slide beneath a table, reach up to the edge, and pull upward while facing upward. As demonstrated in the sample video, an alternative is to utilize a sheet that is securely fastened in a doorway. Leaning back and holding onto the sheet, you drop and then rise yourself again, keeping your arms apart. Work out in as many cycles as possible until you are exhausted. Then, take a 60-second break and repeat the exercise twice more.

The video demo can be accessed at this link: **https://www.youtube.com/watch?v=rloXYB8M3vU**

**Result:**

Trainers recommend horizontal rows as a way to strengthen the arms, shoulders, and core for pull-ups and chin-ups, as well as to help with posture.

# 73

## Reverse Grip Horizontal Row

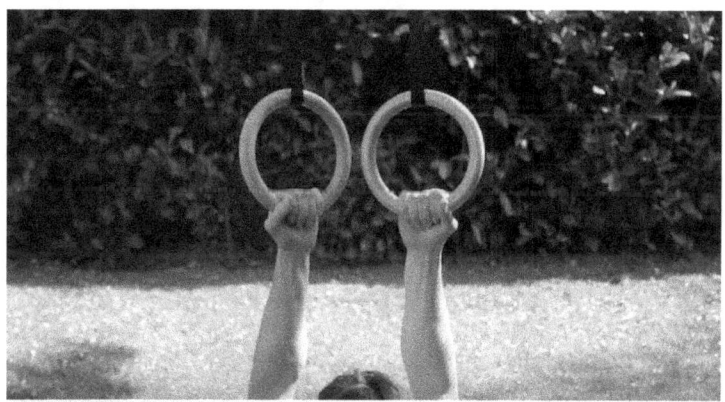

Fig. 13

**Where:**

As you can see in the sample video, this may be done at home or in a training facility where you can grasp onto a bar or a pair of rings.

**How:**

The grasp can be made in two different directions: forward (as seen above) or backward. Additionally, you can have your hands facing either forward or backward. These samples of standard and reverse grips will be shown to you during the demo. To complete a horizontal row, hold onto the ring or bar, bend back, and then straighten up again.

The video demo can be accessed at this link:

**https://www.youtube.com/watch?v=PGcTxvw6-lo**

**Results:**

The muscles of the upper back, particularly the rhomboids, lats, traps, rear delts, and upper arms (particularly the biceps), are developed with reverse and regular horizontal rows.

# 74

# Diamond Push Up

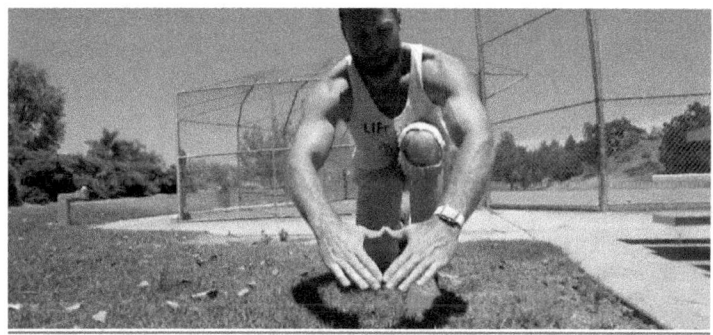

Fig. 14
**Where:**
This exercise can be done on a level, even surface either indoors or outdoors, just like ordinary push-ups.
**How:**
Lie down in a standard push-up position with your arms supporting you and your body fully stretched. Now, instead of putting your hands under your shoulders, move them together

to make a diamond shape with your thumbs and index fingers touching (see above). Put your hands under your sternum by shifting your weight forward.

The video demo can be accessed at this link:
**https://www.youtube.com/watch?v=ZR5U3sb-KeE**
**Results** :

The diamond push-up targets your triceps, delts, and other chest muscles while keeping your hands together and your arms close to your torso.

# 75

## Handstand Push Up

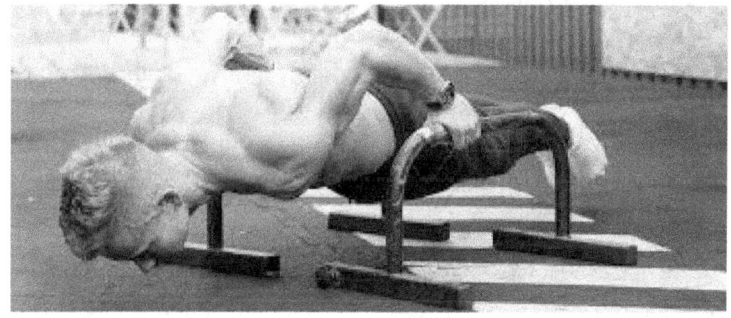

Fig. 15

**Where :**

You can accomplish the handstand push-up outside or indoors using a level surface and two parallel bars as grips. When performing this exercise for the first time, it can be wise to do it near a wall as it can help with balance.

**How:**

This is a tough and demanding workout, but if you push through it and advance step by step, it may be gratifying. You can start with level 1 with your body bent forward and your feet still on the ground, as seen in the image and as you will see in the sample movie. Assume a position so your abs and chest face the wall. You will be putting your feet on the wall for balance and support as you move through the routine's later phases and working your way up to become more vertical. Your ultimate objective will be to push up and down in a vertical, balanced stance without making contact with the wall.

The video demo can be accessed at this link:

**https://www.youtube.com/watch?v=hoHjqYRlXYg**

**Results:**

One of the best workouts for developing your shoulders, upper arms, and triceps is this one. The back in particular is one of the active muscle groups in the core.

# 76

## One-Arm Push-Up/Archer Push

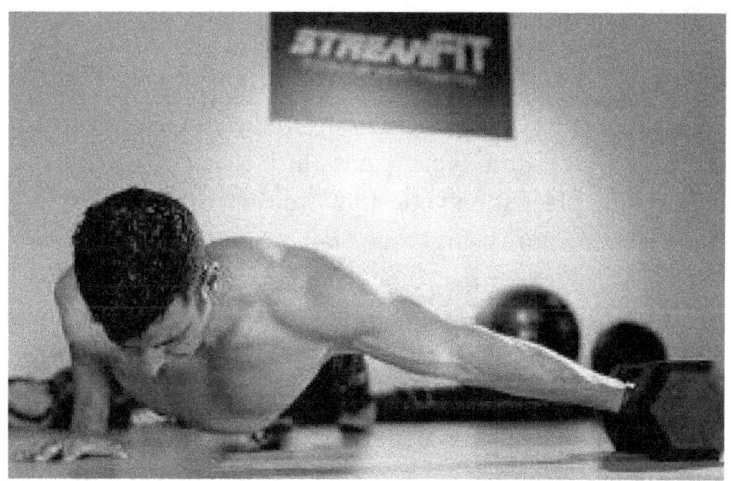

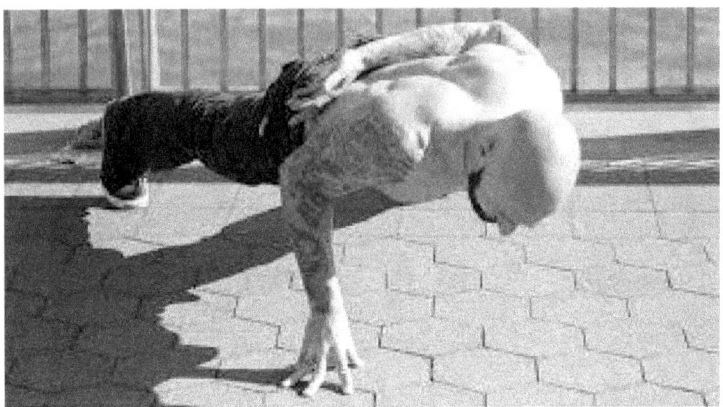

Fig. 16

**Where** :

Any level surface, even a floor, will do.

**How:**

To assist you stay balanced, start in the standard push-up position and then bring your hands a little closer together. Raise an arm and place it on your hips. Lower yourself using just the remaining arm, being careful not to let your body slump or twist. Utilize your arms, shoulders, core, and legs to control the motions. Keep your back straight and not sway. When you descend, avoid twisting your body or lowering your shoulder. Maintain a horizontal body posture.

A version that employs both arms but maintains most of the stress in one is the archer push-up. One arm stays upright, like in the one arm movement, as you can see in the example, but the other arm is extended to the side.

The video demo can be accessed at this link:

**https://www.youtube.com/watch?v=KIEAbfk4cQU**

**Results:**

## ONE-ARM PUSH-UP/ARCHER PUSH

The onearm push-up will provide you a tough, demanding workout once you are able to perform numerous repetitions of the standard push-up. One advantage of unilateral pushups is that they can identify if a person requires compensatory training because one side is weaker than the other. You will need considerably fewer repetitions to reap the benefits of consistent, two-arm push-ups. The arms, shoulders, and entire core will all gain from this.

Straight Bar Dip

77

and Parallel Bars Dip

AND PARALLEL BARS DIP

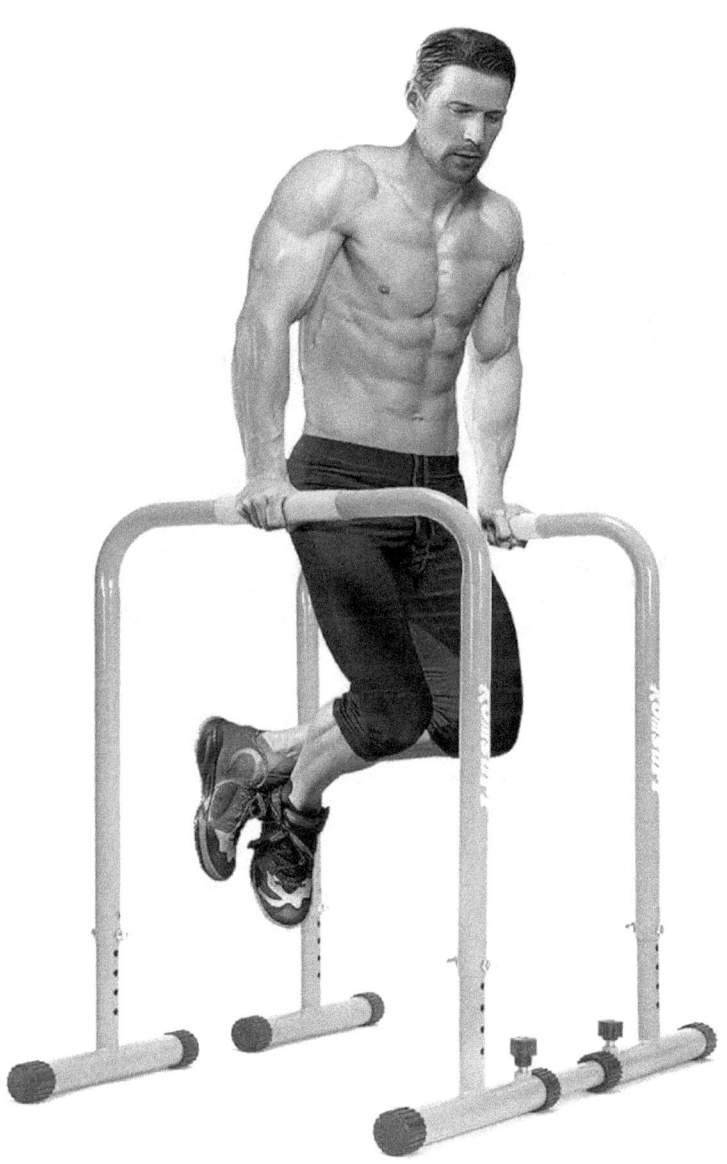

Fig. 17

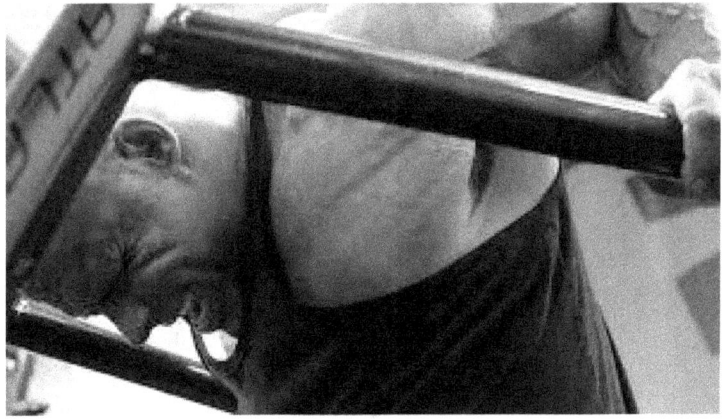

Fig. 18

**Where:**

One (straight) bar or two (parallel) bars are required to conduct dips on a bar.

**How:**

You can either stand between the parallel bars and place one hand on each bar or place your hands on the straight bar to complete the dips. To complete a cycle, push your body weight up until your arms are straight, bend your arms to descend, pause, and then push back up. With a more upright position and a fuller lowering, parallel bar dips are thought to train the muscles, notably the triceps, more correctly. They are also safer and less prone to cause injury. Eight repetitions should be done slowly or as many as you can do without straining yourself too much.

The video demo can be accessed at this link:

**https://www.youtube.com/watch?v=2IUoEAzjZqY**

**Benefits:**

Both parallel bar and straight bar dips work the arms, shoulders, and chest; however, the straight bar dip requires greater internal core rotation and puts more strain on the pectoral (chest) muscles than the parallel bar dip does.

## Tucked Planche Progressions

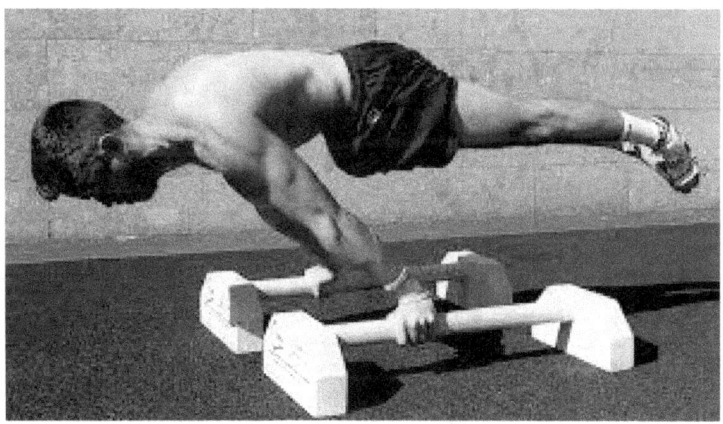

Fig. 19

**Where** :

Similar to floor workouts like push-ups, the tucked planche

can be done on any level surface.

**How** :

Although the tucked planche is sometimes seen as challenging, it can be mastered with the correct setup method. It is worth practicing as part of your advanced levels because it is an excellent calisthenic workout. Warm up by extending one leg and bending toward your knee or bending over and touching your toes to stretch your hamstring muscles. on stretch your core, go on your stomach and raise yourself up using your arms (this is known as the yoga cobra stance). Then, to stretch your lower back, sit back on your heels, bend forward, and extend your arms forward into child's pose. Lean forward, place your hands on the floor, and then stand up again, crouching with your knees wide apart. Roll forward slowly, keeping your elbows inside your knees, until your feet are.

The video demo can be accessed at this link:

**https://www.youtube.com/watch?v=iT1q1Ff02mk**

**Results:**

The core and shoulders benefit greatly from the tucked planche. In addition, it strengthens the chest, triceps, and serratus anterior muscles, all of which contribute to better posture.

AND PARALLEL BARS DIP

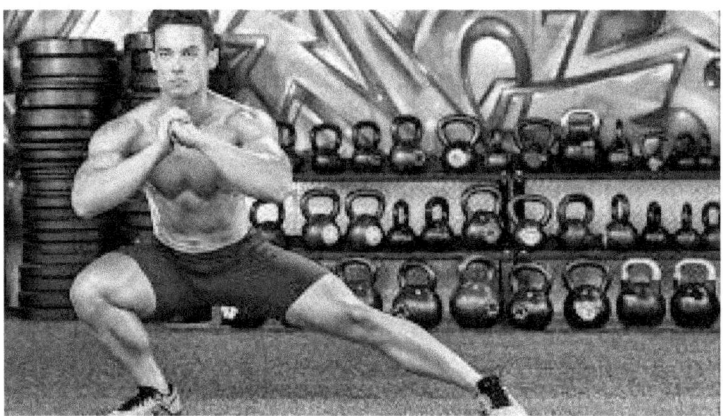

Lateral Lunge
Fig. 20
**Where:**
You can practice lateral lunges outside or on a flat surface, but make sure there's enough room for you to take big steps sideways.
**How:**
Place your feet about eighteen inches apart and stand straight. Step three steps to the left with your left leg, then squat down on your right leg. Remain centered with your weight on your glutes. After a brief pause, raise yourself back up to the upright position. On the left side, repeat the motion. Throughout the workout, keep your body upright to maintain your balance. Start with eight repetitions and work your way up to twelve as you advance. Work out in two or three sets, taking a 60-second break in between.
The video demo can be accessed at this link:
**https://www.youtube.com/watch?v=gwWv7aPcD88**
**Results:**

A basic yet powerful exercise for building quadriceps, glutes, and hip flexors is the lateral lunge. As your strategy gets underway, you can encounter certain issues. Which is why the next chapter will cover some common questions and troubleshooting concerns that you may run into when you work through your bodyweight calisthenics program.

## Chapter 8
### Troubleshooting

The goal of this chapter is to foresee your potential concerns and difficulties and offer answers and solutions. As with any instructional book, there may be questions that come up that are not covered in the explanations and directions. Let's review some foundational knowledge before we get started in order to allay your worries.

### First, Do No Harm

Exercises involving bodyweight calisthenics are thought to be safer and less likely to result in damage than weightlifting, although pulls, tears, and strains from overuse should not be taken lightly. Keep an eye on your body and avoid going overboard. Take it easy and don't push yourself to perform the pushups in agony if you are attempting to complete 12 and finding it difficult to get past number eight if your shoulders are screaming in pain. This time, you might have ran out of energy, even if you had completed 12 reps a few days prior or during a previous set. That's alright, too. You might be able to return to 12 reps with just a few days of recuperation. Consider it this way:

It's critical to avoid pushing yourself past your physical

limitations. This can be achieved by exercising incorrectly, doing too many repetitions, skipping breaks between sets, not giving yourself two full days to recover between workouts, or adopting a position that places an intolerable amount of strain on a ligament, muscle, or joint.

### You Are Unique

Except for identical twins, no two individuals have the same DNA, which implies that no two persons are alike in terms of abilities, talents, capacities, and stamina. Everybody has unique mental and cognitive abilities. Therefore, we shouldn't hold ourselves to the same standards as others. We used statistics and the knowledge of numerous coaches, trainers, and sports medicine specialists to determine the Basic, Intermediate, and Advanced levels for reps, sets, cycle speeds, and rest intervals between sets. However, they are not strict requirements that you must fulfill; rather, they are merely estimations designed to help. Your physiology will determine how you develop muscles with both bulk and definition. You ought to honor the unique characteristics of your body. Rest certain that if you labor at this.

### Give Your Muscles Time to Build

It takes time for your muscles to repair after intense exercise damages their cells and fibers. After a strenuous workout, you could feel "pumped up" and muscular, but that's just the blood and other fluids temporarily collecting; it will go away in a few hours. You shouldn't expect your muscles to grow to an enormous size in a matter of days because the actual growth of muscle tissue occurs slowly and at the microscopic level. However, the development of your lower body, core, and upper body muscles will show over the course of several weeks and months. Give it time.

Bodyweight Calisthenics Q&As

Now that we've covered the introduction, here are the responses to some of your more specific queries.

**Q:** Are calisthenics effective exercises for fitness?

**A:** Except for a bar for pull-ups, chin-ups, and rows, calisthenics is a unique and acknowledged type of physical training intended to develop strength and muscle using only one's own bodyweight as an alternative to weights, machines, and other equipment. Strength, definition, and bulk can all be added to muscle with calisthenics. However, in contrast to some other types of exercise, it also helps you become more functional and flexible because it doesn't make you tight, muscle-bound, or inflexible. Exercises involving calisthenics are portable and simple to learn. Do not undervalue the benefits of using your own bodyweight or the simplicity and accessibility of calisthenics as a means of building a fantastic physique. Even at a just ninety pounds, you will.

**Q:** Do I need to do any special training before beginning bodyweight calisthenics?

**A:** Should you be in a pretty decent health, you should be able to start exercising right now, if you so choose. To ensure that you progress at a reasonable rate, the Basic amount plans purposefully start you off with a low amount of repetitions and progressively increase reps and shorten rest periods. See your doctor if you're not sure if your health can handle the task; they might recommend a physical examination. This is particularly crucial if you're just starting out with cardiovascular activity.

**Q:** Is it true that calisthenics builds muscle?

**A:** The answer is definitely "yes" when it comes to bodyweight calisthenics as they are described in this book. Some people think of calisthenics as cardio exercises, jumping jacks, skipping rope, and stretching. However, bodyweight exercises like calisthenics are a very safe, affordable, and efficient approach to gain muscle for more definition and bulk. Bodyweight resistance causes the process known as hypertrophy, which results in more muscle tissue being repaired than destroyed and leads to muscle growth. Hypertrophy is caused by physical tension and metabolic stress that destroys muscle fibers and cells.

**Q:** Is exercising with bodyweight calisthenics superior than training with weights?

**A:** No, it's just not the same. However, there is no superiority between weight training and calisthenics. Building muscle and strength are the main objectives of both bodyweight calisthenics and weightlifting. You may gain muscle mass a little bit quicker by using resistance training equipment and lifting weights, which are particularly good at causing hypertrophy. However, that is countered by the fact that calisthenics don't require access to a gym or training facility and are less likely to result in damage. Some skilled practitioners of calisthenics will incorporate resistance equipment and weights into their exercises. For instance, squat while grasping a barbell or a set of dumbbells. We advise you to start with just calisthenics, and if you keep upping the reps, decreasing the cycle periods, and cutting down on the rest in between sets, you.

**Q:** How frequently should I work out?

**A:** You should prioritize giving yourself enough time to recuperate between workouts, as we covered in chapters 6 and 7. It was shown that this should be at least two rest days. There are two possibilities for scheduling the exercises in the 21-day plans: either complete all nine calisthenics exercises in one session (called "nine-in-one"), or do part of the set of exercises one day and the rest the next day (called "nine-in-two"). Either way, the working muscles are not activated and tested again until after two days of rest.

If your workout is on Monday, for instance, you would recover and perform no bodyweight calisthenics on Tuesday or Wednesday and then resume all nine exercises on Thursday if you follow the nine-in-one program. It's acceptable to space out your calisthenics routines by three days. However, avoid taking too long breaks between workouts since this may cause you to lose strength and make it harder to resume the exercise. In conclusion, two or three times a week of training should be dedicated to each muscle group.

**Q:** Is it possible to combine cardiovascular exercises with bodyweight calisthenics in one day?

**A:** Yes, it is a common practice, particularly when both are carried out in the same establishment, such as a gym or fitness center. Many feel that "getting it all done" in one long session is both convenient and enjoyable. The enhanced flow of beta-endorphins is another reason for the satisfaction. Cardio and weight training together have a cumulative, or synergistic, effect where the whole is equal to or greater than the sum of its parts. The majority of individuals who enjoy both types of exercise choose to perform their cardio first and then their calisthenics right after. Why? While calisthenics enhances circulation to the targeted muscle region, cardio warms the body as a whole by improving circulation to almost every cell and muscle.

**Q:** Injured or in pain, should I still work out?

**A:** The short response is no. First, do no harm, as we stated at the beginning of this chapter (this phrase is taken from the Hippocratic oath that physicians must pronounce in order to obtain a license to practice medicine). It is important to emphasize again, though, that pushing yourself while you are truly in pain is not beneficial and is a sign that you are hurt or about to get hurt. Try to gradually alleviate any discomfort you get in your muscles or joints by assessing whether it's something you can handle, something that needs to be rested, or something more serious that needs to be checked out by a medical professional.

Nevertheless, it's critical to identify and learn how to manage minor discomforts like soreness, stiffness, or muscle burn from exercise.

**Q:** Will doing calisthenics aid in my weight loss?

**A:** If your caloric expenditure exceeds your caloric intake, weight loss is likely to occur. This basic scientific principle has no exceptions or short cuts. Because each person has a different metabolism—the rate at which their body uses energy—no two people burn calories at the same pace. It is therefore possible for two people following the same diet and exercise regimen to experience different weight gains or decreases.

A quality calisthenics workout will typically burn between 200 and 400 calories. Over the course of a few weeks, incorporating calisthenics movements into your regimen while maintaining the same level of physical activity might result in as much as.

However, there are a few more things to think about. Since muscle is denser than the fat it is replacing, more muscle mass might result in an increase in weight. Your metabolism slows down after exercising, especially when you're at rest, so your daily net calorie loss may be less than you initially anticipated. This applies to both aerobic and calisthenics exercises. The most efficient strategy to lose weight is to combine exercise with calorie reduction in your diet. To discuss the best sources of calories, see the section on nutrition and the Mediterranean diet in chapter 2.

**Q:** What happens if the Basic or Intermediate 21-Day Plans don't allow me to complete every rep?

**A:** You should follow your individual talents and perform the number of repetitions for each exercise that pushes you, but you should also know when to quit. As previously mentioned, the programs are recommendations based on averages and significant experience. Generally speaking, eight to twelve reps should be the optimal number, with the final two feeling extremely difficult but manageable without compromising form. Push-ups performed without lowering all the way down are examples of bad form, as is kicking your way toward the chin-up bar. whether deciding whether to end, refer to the "last two" instances of toughness. You should stop there if you are struggling to finish rep number eight with proper form and without doing the movement carelessly.

**Q:** What happens if there aren't enough representatives in the plans? Is there anything else I can do?

**A:** As previously stated, you should respect your own abilities and the 21-day programs are suggestions rather than strict guidelines. You have three choices to think about if the quantity of repetitions is insufficient to get you to the "last two" difficult rounds:

**Do more reps.** Just make sure you're doing all the repetitions correctly—that is, with complete ups and downs, a straight back, and proper form and posture. Make sure you are not cutting corners as well.

**Shorten the rest time between sets.** Reduce the 60-second rest period between sets, for instance, to 30 seconds. When you take fewer breaks between sets, you should notice that the repetitions become harder.

**Slow the cycle rate of each rep so that each movement takes longer.**

For instance, slowing down and requiring 10 seconds to do a pull-up or chin-up, or needing 12 seconds to complete one push-up cycle.

Q: What happens if I don't get the desired outcome?

A: First, read through the sections labeled "You are Unique" and "Give Your Muscles Time to Build" at the beginning of this chapter. These clarify why you have to be patient before achieving the desired outcomes and how your body develops muscles at a different rate. This is not to say, however, that you should give up on your goals of having a toned body and increased strength. Even if it can take longer than you anticipate, the sequence of 21-day regimens will undoubtedly get you there. The most crucial thing is to try your best to adhere to the programs, putting in the effort during each calisthenics session and making sure you give yourself enough time to rest and recover in between workouts. Additionally, you want to confirm that you've.

Things You Might Be Doing Wrong

There are a few more things that can be impeding your efforts to gain muscle and strength. Diet, sleep, stress, and both excessive and insufficient labor are a few of them.

1. **Protein**

Diet was covered in the section above, but now let's concentrate on protein. Do you get adequate nourishment? Although meat is one of the best sources of protein, we are advised to limit our intake of red meat for cardiovascular health, so it can be challenging. However, that speaks of beef that has been heavily marbled with saturated fats. Limit your intake to lean, low-fat, or fat-free portions of chicken, turkey, beef, and pork. Before cooking, trim off any visible fat. Eat fish at least twice a week to reap the benefits of its even better quality protein along with other nutrients and antioxidants.

But beyond meat and fish, there are other valuable sources of protein. Select beans, healthy grains, nuts, and veggies that are strong in protein. Add eggs and low-fat or fat-free dairy to your diet as well. Choose the Greek or Icelandic yogurt varieties if you enjoy yogurt, as they have a high protein content (18 to 19 grams per ¾ cup serving).

1. **Sleep**

Do you get enough sleep each night to allow your body to heal itself?

Everybody requires a restful night's sleep. Our brains must first process all of the information and impressions from the day by allowing our 100 billion neurons to reorganize their trillions of neural connections and saturating the cells and neurons with enzymes and cleansing fluids that eliminate potentially harmful waste products and plaques that may impair cognitive function. We require the time we dream to further organize and purge our memories and thoughts. Furthermore, a large portion of the healing and reconstruction of our injured muscles occurs when we sleep. This is the best period because the muscles are not used and there will be less disruptions to the healing process. However, if you don't receive the necessary.

It is worthwhile to consider this: Poor sleep habits cause all that hard work doing calisthenics to be stopped, as well as the necessary rebuilding. Refer to the chapter 3 section on sleep and keep in mind that eight hours of sleep every night is optimal. Make a note of the techniques that will enable you to get to sleep and remain asleep. Set aside time specifically to go to bed and wake up at the same times each day. Additionally, keep electronic devices out of the bedroom!

1. **Stress**

Do you still feel anxious or stressed out about your life?

It occurs to everyone. Stress is essentially the central nervous system's self-defense mechanism and is a typical response to danger or risk. The well-known fight-or-flight response of the sympathetic nervous system is triggered, resulting in blood pressure rises, rapid heartbeat, and increases in the chemicals cortisol and adrenaline (which deliver glycogen to the muscles for an instant energy boost). However, this reaction is intended to be a temporary emergency remedy. Once the threat has passed, it ought to completely disappear. However, stress becomes chronic much too often. In severe circumstances, your body's ability to rebuild itself may be compromised, which could slow down or even prevent you from gaining muscle.

4. **Too Little or Too Much**

Do you exercise too little or too much?

It's possible that you are underexercising, which is keeping you from reaching your goals of developing muscle. The 21-day regimens are made to strengthen your muscles:

➢ in the appropriate number of sets

➢ with the appropriate amount of rest in between sets

➢ with the necessary rest and recovery time in between workouts

➢ at the appropriate frequency (reps)

➢ at the appropriate pace (cycles)

Muscular growth will be delayed to occur or may not occur at all if you are not making an effort to at least moderately follow the programs. There is no place in life where the adage "You get out of it what you put into it" is more true. Everyone experiences sluggish days or misses the odd workout, but if you are willing to put in the effort, you can have a fantastic body.

You can do this, I promise. Excessive exercise has negative effects on its own. Your muscles may become irreparably damaged by frequent and excessive exercise, making them unrepairable with rest and recuperation. Moreover, rather than gaining mass, power, and definition.

You can do this, I promise. Excessive exercise has negative effects on its own. Your muscles may become irreparably damaged by frequent and excessive exercise, making them unrepairable with rest and recuperation. In addition, your muscles may atrophy, or lose size and strength, rather of gaining mass, power, and strength. Adhere to the schedule; if there's anything that should come first, it's the days off and recuperation in between sessions. Allow your body the time it needs to recover so that the damaged muscle fibers may be rebuilt. Avoid rushing into the advanced levels too soon and stick to the rep, set, and cycle speed limits that are suggested in the 21-day schedules.

# 78

# Myths and Misconceptions

You might not know what is real and what is a myth or misconception with everything that is written in periodicals, on social media, and in advertisements, not to mention what you might hear others saying in gyms and fitness facilities. These are ten of the most widespread misconceptions around fitness and calisthenics, along with the information you need to dispel them:

**Myth 1:** Your muscles will become larger the more and harder you train. Feeling both anxious and excited is normal. Now that your calisthenics bodybuilding program is underway and going well, why not increase the frequency and intensity of your workouts to get better, faster results? Although the answer is obvious from the other chapters, let me reiterate: Your muscles won't grow if you overuse them and don't give them adequate time to recuperate between workouts; in fact, this could cause atrophy or loss of muscular mass. Moreover, pushing yourself too far can lead to accidents. Adhere to the 21-day plans' pace and refrain from overworking and understretching your muscles.

**Myth 2:** Daily soreness should follow each calisthenics session. While some soreness the day after a workout is common and usually not cause for alarm, it might serve as a nice reminder that you worked out hard the day before. However, pain that is severe, uncomfortable, or persistent (lasting more than two or three days) indicates that you are working too hard, performing too many repetitions, or not resting enough between sets. Muscle pain should only occur sometimes as you condition; it shouldn't be severe or persistent. Keep an eye out for any joint soreness and make sure you're doing every exercise correctly.

**Myth 3:**

Taking vitamins is more crucial than your diet. There is no precedent for us to disregard a healthy, balanced diet in favor of attempting to obtain our nutrients from highly processed, extremely concentrated supplements, as humans have developed over many thousands of years by eating a diversity of natural, unprocessed foods. A product that makes exaggerated and deceptive claims about providing faster-growing, more muscular muscles is not what it seems.

Since obtaining 100 grams of protein from diet alone can be challenging, you might want to look into whey protein supplements; nevertheless, a high-quality diet should always come first. Supermarkets also sell food-based smoothies and beverages that include 20 to 30 grams of protein. (The complete overview of nutrition is provided in chapter 2.)

**Myth 4:**

Your muscle turns to fat when your workouts halt or slow down.

Nine of the 20 amino acids that make up protein, the complex chemical that makes up muscle, are exclusively found in food. Muscle fibers repair themselves by utilizing protein and amino acids when we exercise and cause damage to them. The size of our muscles will gradually decrease if we start to slow down or even stop working out. Since fat is primarily made up of free fatty acids, it is physically impossible for muscle to convert to fat. However, weight gain results from a pause in exercise and an increase in calorie intake, which is then stored as fat in the body.

**Myth 5:**

By strengthening your core, particularly your abs, you can lose belly fat. Exercises targeting the core will help to define and harden the muscles in the abdomen, but it is not possible to burn off fat deposits or "spot reduce" it. Losing weight is the only way to remove the fat from your stomach and expose the six-pack that lies beneath it. And the greatest approach to lose weight consistently is to pair your bodyweight calisthenics exercises with a sensible diet that lowers your intake of calories and food, particularly processed carbohydrates. Additionally, to grow muscle and feel filled for longer, limit your intake of fats, steer clear of sugar and other empty calories, and increase the amount of protein in your diet.

**Myth 6:**

Seniors shouldn't work out too frequently or too hard. Exercise is beneficial to people of all ages, but it becomes even more important as people age. Your heart is one of the muscles that benefit from exercise. You may keep your heart strong and your arteries open by getting your heart to pump harder by gently warming up, then increasing to a steady, rhythmic rate and sustaining it for 20, 30, or more minutes, many days a week (or more). As outlined in our 21-day regimens, calisthenics will help you develop and retain strength, increase flexibility, and reduce your risk of injury. Additionally, cardio exercising will improve heart health.

**Myth 7:**

Large muscles cannot be built with calisthenics. Everything here hinges on your definition of large muscles. If you want to appear like an Olympic weightlifter, you will need to train like one as well, using extremely high weights over a period of years that will be, to put it mildly, harsh. But calisthenics is the best workout regimen for you if your objective is to have the well-developed muscular size, definition, and strength of an athlete. Look at Olympic gymnasts instead to understand where a quality calisthenics program may take you.

**Myth 8:**

Only specific body types can benefit from calisthenics.

It's a common fallacy that persons with thin physiques benefit more from calisthenics than those with larger or heavier frames. Although different body types adapt and develop muscle in different ways, calisthenics can be beneficial for all body types. Although they don't usually add much bulk, lightweight constructions seem to produce the gymnast's physique and good definition more quickly. Because their increased body weight provides more resistance, heavier builds gain strength and bulk more quickly. Since most of us fall somewhere in the middle, calisthenics can help us gain both good definition and muscle mass.

**Myth 9:**

The most crucial place to develop is the upper body. Seeing large shoulders, triceps, biceps, and, of course, well-developed upper chest pectoral muscles, impresses us all. However, you should concentrate on training your entire body because the muscles in your lower body and core are just as important, if not more so. The muscles of the back, lower back, and abdomen make up the core. Strong core muscles improve overall strength and reduce the risk of injury. Since your hip flexors, quadriceps, hamstrings, and calves support and propel you forward for an average of almost 2,000 kilometers each year, you should also work on strengthening them.

**Myth 10:**

It's not necessary to perform every exercise with flawless technique in order to gain muscle mass and strength.

# 79

# Conclusion

The goal of this book is to assist anyone, regardless of ability level, in achieving their ideal muscular physique and overall physical state. You have committed to and invested in yourself by choosing to study and use the advice in this book, so congrats on making this crucial first move. Recognize that:

➤ Although you've never had the motivation or time to work toward it in the past, you've promised yourself that you will ultimately have the physique of your dreams.

➤ You see that achieving your goals can be done in less than an hour, in as few as three days a week.

➤ You are free to take up the task.

➤ By making the biggest investment of your life, you are extending your life and improving your strength and health.

➤ You're on the right track to perform the bodyweight calisthenics exercises that have been hand-picked for optimal results; 21-day plans consist of just nine exercises that will take you from beginner to expert, assisting you in building strong muscle at every level.

➤ You are aware of the importance of two.

## CONCLUSION

Never undervalue your abilities. You are stronger than you know, in spite of whatever questions or worries you may have. And right now, you're going to get stronger, gain more defined muscles, and experience a significant increase in your general physical capacity. It is absolutely your right to get stronger and more attractive. You should feel physically and mentally well so that you may develop self-worth and the confidence that comes from knowing you can do everything you set your mind to.

Knowing that you possess the physical power and endurance of a well-trained athlete, you may anticipate the respect and support of others, who will look to you for leadership. The moment is drawing near when you will be able to declare, no matter the difficulty:

**"I can handle this. I have command of the circumstance. I'll finish it.**

To help us ensure that this is the best source of instruction and encouragement for everyone looking to build bigger muscles and increase their strength through bodyweight calisthenics, we would appreciate your honest opinion on this book. In order to let others know that this is the perfect book for them, please give us a five-star review if this book met or surpassed your expectations.

To help us ensure that this is the best source of instruction and encouragement for everyone looking to build bigger muscles and increase their strength through bodyweight calisthenics, we would appreciate your honest opinion on this book. In order to let others know that this is the perfect book for them, please give us a five-star review if this book met or surpassed your expectations. We wish you well, prosperity, and personal fulfillment. But first, think about and accept what we know to be beyond a shadow of a doubt:

"That is definitely something—you are tougher, fitter, and stronger than you were when you first started!"
- **Daily Jay**

## WRITTEN BY:
## ALLANA ROBSON


## THANK YOU

www.ingramcontent.com/pod-product-compliance
Lightning Source LLC
LaVergne TN
LVHW011943070526
838202LV00054B/4771